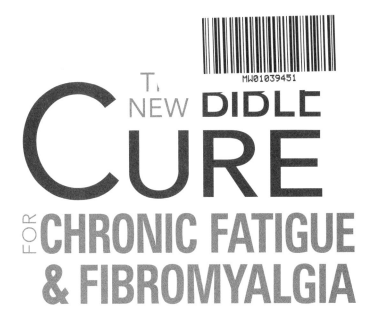

THE NEW BIBLE CURE FOR CHRONIC FATIGUE & FIBROMYALGIA

DON COLBERT, MD

SILOAM

Most CHARISMA HOUSE BOOK GROUP products are available at special quantity discounts for bulk purchase for sales promotions, premiums, fund-raising, and educational needs. For details, write Charisma House Book Group, 600 Rinehart Road, Lake Mary, Florida 32746, or telephone (407) 333-0600.

THE NEW BIBLE CURE FOR CHRONIC FATIGUE AND FIBROMYALGIA by Don Colbert, MD
Published by Siloam
Charisma Media/Charisma House Book Group
600 Rinehart Road
Lake Mary, Florida 32746
www.charismahouse.com

All Scripture quotations are from the Holy Bible, New Living Translation, copyright © 1996, 2004. Used by permission of Tyndale House Publishers, Inc., Wheaton, IL 60189. All rights reserved.

Scripture quotations marked NKJV are from the New King James Version of the Bible. Copyright © 1979, 1980, 1982 by Thomas Nelson, Inc., publishers. Used by permission.

Cover design by Nathan Morgan
Design Director: Bill Johnson

Visit the author's website at www.drcolbert.com.

Library of Congress Cataloging-in-Publication Data:
Colbert, Don.
  The new Bible cure for chronic fatigue and fibromyalgia / Don Colbert.
-- [Rev. and updated].
      p. cm.
  Rev. ed. of: The Bible cure for chronic fatigue and fibromyalgia.
  Includes bibliographical references (p.   ).
  ISBN 978-1-59979-867-7 (trade paper) -- ISBN 978-1-61638-430-2
(e-book) 1. Fibromyalgia--Religious aspects--Christianity. 2.
Fibromyalgia--Alternative treatment. 3. Fibromyalgia--Popular works. 4.

Chronic fatigue syndrome--Religious aspects--Christianity. 5. Chronic
fatigue syndrome--Alternative treatment. 6. Chronic fatigue
syndrome--Popular works. I. Colbert, Don. Bible cure for chronic
fatigue and fibromyalgia. II. Title.

RC927.3.C65 2011
616.7'42--dc22

2011013624

CONTENTS

A BRAND-NEW BIBLE CURE
FOR A BRAND-NEW YOU!

I F YOU ARE often overwhelmed by fatigue that saps your strength and robs your life—fatigue that will simply not go away even with adequate rest—you are not alone. According to a recent article in *The Pain Practitioner*, a publication of the American Academy of Pain Management, at least one million Americans suffer from chronic fatigue syndrome. More than 80 percent of those cases are undiagnosed despite the fact that people are experiencing extreme fatigue.[1] "For years, this medical condition has been marginalized and misunderstood," says Kim Kenney, executive director of the Chronic Fatigue and Immune Dysfunction Association of America.[2]

Many individuals with chronic fatigue also have fibromyalgia. The two disorders have been described as "separate but related." In fibromyalgia, musculoskeletal pain accompanies chronic fatigue. As you'll see in the coming pages, sleep disturbances are often at the root of both the fatigue and pain experienced by sufferers, and I will address these and other issues throughout this book.

As a Christian medical doctor I've studied and prayed about the causes of disease, and increasingly I've discovered that many diseases have very strong spiritual, mental, and emotional roots. If you are familiar with my books, then doubtless you are aware that I believe in the health of the entire person: body, mind, and spirit.

Although traditional medicine often sees these facets of our beings as very separate, in truth they are not. A vital link exists between the spirit, soul, and body. And although much of the disease and physical pain we suffer comes from the body, often these distresses begin in the soul, which encompasses the mind, will, and emotions.

Therefore, truly living in the divine health that God intends for us requires that we look a little deeper, beyond the physical process of disease to the spiritual, emotional, and mental roots. I trust that you will find these pages extremely enlightening as you gain new insight and revelation to help you live your life in the robust, joyful, peaceful state of good health that God desires for you.

By picking up this Bible Cure book, you have taken an exciting first step toward successfully conquering chronic fatigue syndrome and fibromyalgia and reclaiming control over your spiritual, emotional, and physical health. Right now you may be confronting some of the greatest challenges of your life. But by understanding some of the "real" root causes of your chronic fatigue and fibromyalgia, you can rise to a new level of physical, emotional, and spiritual health and joy in God.

Jesus Christ promises you rest, refreshment, restoration, and renewal. He said, "Come to me, all of you who are weary and carry heavy burdens, and I will give you rest. Take my yoke upon you. Let me teach you, because I am humble and gentle at heart, and you will find rest for your souls" (Matt. 11:28–29).

Chronic fatigue and fibromyalgia are not God's plan for you. His Word promises, "'For I know the plans I have for you,' says the LORD. 'They are plans for good and not for disaster, to give you a future and a hope. In those days when you pray, I will listen. If you look for me wholeheartedly, you will find me. I will be found by you'" (Jer. 29:11–14). So you see, God desires that you conquer your fatigue and discover power and energy to live life to the fullest.

BE ENCOURAGED AND ENERGIZED!

So as you read this book, get ready to defeat the symptoms of chronic fatigue syndrome and fibromyalgia. You will begin to feel better physically, emotionally, and spiritually. This Bible Cure book is filled with practical steps, hope, encouragement, and valuable information on how to stay fit and healthy. Originally published as *The Bible Cure for Chronic Fatigue and Fibromyalgia* in 2000, *The New Bible Cure for Chronic Fatigue and Fibromyalgia* has been revised and updated with the latest medical research on these two closely related conditions. If you compare this book side by side with the previous edition, you'll see that it's also larger, allowing me to expand greatly upon the information provided in the previous edition and provide you with a deeper understanding of what you face and how to overcome it.

Unchanged from the previous edition are the timeless, life-changing, and healing scriptures throughout this book that will strengthen and encourage your spirit and soul. The proven principles, truths, and guidelines in these passages anchor the practical and medical insights also contained in this book. They will effectively focus your prayers, thoughts, and actions so you can step into God's plan of divine health for you—a plan that includes victory over chronic fatigue and fibromyalgia.

Another change since the original *The Bible Cure for Chronic Fatigue and Fibromyalgia* was published is that I've released a book called *The Seven Pillars of Health*. I encourage you to read it because the principles of health it contains are the foundation to healthy living that will affect all areas of your life. It sets the stage for everything you will ever read in any other book I've published—including this one.

There is much you can do to prevent or overcome your

symptoms. The Bible Cure plan will energize you with confidence, determination, and knowledge to live victoriously. God's healing power is greater than any fatigue and pain that you now face. You no longer have to be weary and burdened. The Bible Cure promise for you is this:

> He gives power to the weak and strength to the powerless.
>
> —ISAIAH 40:29

It is my prayer that the power of faith in God's wonderful Word and the divine touch of His healing hand, together with practical suggestions for health, nutrition, and fitness in this book, will restore your health, energy, vitality, and joy!

—DON COLBERT, MD

A **BIBLE CURE** Prayer for You

Almighty God, You are the source of all power and strength. You have said that You give Your people strength. So I ask You to break the spirit of heaviness and weariness in my body and give me the knowledge and wisdom to eat correctly and to live well. Help me overcome fatigue and pain and become energized to serve and worship You with my whole heart, mind, body, and strength. Empower me to accomplish Your purpose and plans for my life. In You I will find my rest and strength. Amen.

Chapter 1

UNDERSTANDING CHRONIC FATIGUE AND FIBROMYALGIA

A N ANCIENT AND powerful biblical proverb reads, "If a bird sees a trap being set, it knows to stay away" (Prov. 1:17). That means an enemy cannot trap you if you can see and understand what he is doing. If your enemy is chronic fatigue syndrome or fibromyalgia, then according to the proverb, your first step to victory is to understand these conditions.

Armed with factual, truthful knowledge about what you are facing, you will better know how to pray and make wise treatment decisions. God does not intend for you to accept passively the physical attacks that assault you. You can fight back with knowledge, wisdom, faith, and prayer! In the natural you can strengthen your immune system, and in the spiritual realm, you can strengthen your faith.

Make this scripture prayer your own Bible Cure prayer as you read this chapter and develop both natural and spiritual insight about your condition:

> You are my strength; I wait for you to rescue me, for you, O God, are my fortress.... O my Strength, to you I sing praises, for you, O God, are my refuge, the God who shows me unfailing love.
>
> —PSALM 59:9, 17

UNDERSTANDING THE BATTLE

Chronic fatigue syndrome (CFS), also called chronic fatigue and immune dysfunction syndrome (CFIDS), is a severe, incapacitating fatigue that isn't improved by adequate rest. In spite of more than twenty-five years of research, there is no known cure for CFS. It is usually accompanied by an entire host of debilitating symptoms and is diagnosed when these symptoms and the fatigue have lasted at least six months with no other explanation for their cause.

Symptoms include debilitating fatigue that is not improved by bed rest and may be worsened by physical or mental activity, sleep difficulties (trouble falling asleep or staying asleep), impairment of short-term memory or concentration, sore throat, tender lymph nodes in the neck and armpits, muscle and joint pain without redness or swelling, and headaches. Additional symptoms include blurry vision, eye pain, or light sensitivity; gastrointestinal disturbances; chills and night sweats; allergies and sensitivities to foods, odors, chemicals, and medications; irritability, mood swings, anxiety, and panic attacks; difficulty maintaining upright posture, dizziness, balance problems, and fainting; and gynecological problems such as PMS and endometriosis.

CFS affects different people in varying degrees, but all individuals with CFS function at a substantially lower level of activity than before onset of the illness. Some are able to continue holding jobs, attending school, or caring for themselves or family members.[1] Others are profoundly affected by it. About 25 percent of people suffering from CFS are fully disabled by the disorder.[2]

CFS is not a disease; it is a syndrome, which means it is a group of related symptoms without a known physical cause. It is often diagnosed in conjunction with other syndromes that share some of its symptoms, such as fibromyalgia, irritable bowel syndrome

(IBS), postural orthostatic tachycardia syndrome (POTS), neurally mediated hypotension (NMH), temporomandibular joint disorder (TMJ), multiple chemical sensitivities (MCS), and others. We will focus mainly on chronic fatigue and fibromyalgia in this book, since the symptoms and treatments of these two syndromes are so similar.

Take this self-test to help assess whether or not you are experiencing the symptoms of chronic fatigue syndrome.

A BIBLE CURE *Health Tip*

Has your activity level been reduced by 50 percent in the past six months because of fatigue that seemed to come on all at once? If other fatigue-causing illnesses have been factored out, this is the major criterion for diagnosing chronic fatigue syndrome. Check the common symptoms of chronic fatigue syndrome that you are experiencing. If you are experiencing eight of these minor criteria symptoms, then ask your doctor to examine you for chronic fatigue syndrome.

- ❏ Mild fever
- ❏ Recurrent sore throat
- ❏ Painful lymph nodes
- ❏ Muscle weakness
- ❏ Muscle pain
- ❏ Prolonged fatigue after exercise
- ❏ Recurrent headache
- ❏ Migratory joint pains
- ❏ Neurological or psychological complaints
- ❏ Sensitivity to bright light
- ❏ Forgetfulness
- ❏ Confusion

❏ Inability to concentrate
❏ Excessive irritability
❏ Depression
❏ Sleep disturbance (either sleeping too much or an inability to sleep)

If you are experiencing symptoms of chronic fatigue, get a complete physical exam by your medical doctor and a thorough evaluation by a nutritional doctor.

Your doctor will need to rule out a number of diseases that are also linked to excessive fatigue. In addition, chronic fatigue can also be a side effect of certain medications, including antihistamines, blood pressure medications, arthritis medications, antianxiety medications, tranquilizers, antidepressants, and numerous other medications.

As I mentioned earlier, fibromyalgia shares many of the same symptoms and remedies as chronic fatigue syndrome, but it has some additional factors as well. Let's take a look.

FIBROMYALGIA

Fibromyalgia is a rheumatologic disorder that most commonly affects women but also strikes men and children of all ethnic backgrounds. If you are experiencing this condition, your fatigue accompanies widespread musculoskeletal pain and trigger points (extremely tender points) in specific areas of the body.

Eighteen different trigger points for fibromyalgia have been identified. These include the muscles in the neck, in the upper back (including trapezius muscles), in the mid-back, at the base of the skull, in the buttocks, in the upper portion of the thigh and the lateral thigh, just above the lateral elbow, and in the rib cage, especially around the second rib, as well as others.

The major symptoms include:

- Pain in at least eleven of the trigger points of the body when a specified amount of pressure is applied
- Muscle aches, pain, and stiffness in arms, legs, and trunk for at least three months

The minor symptoms include:

- Sleep disturbances
- Irritable bowel syndrome
- Temporomandibular joint disorder (TMJ) symptoms
- Chronic headache
- Tingling sensations or numbness
- Swelling of the joints
- Depression, anxiety, irritability, or decreased memory
- Symptoms varying in intensity with activity, stress, or changes in weather

Disorders that produce similar symptoms to the above must be excluded before an official diagnosis can be made. Since people with fibromyalgia appear healthy and conventional medical tests such as X-rays and blood tests usually do not reveal any abnormalities, it's important to visit a doctor who is knowledgeable about fibromyalgia, such as a rheumatologist, if you think you may be dealing with this condition.

GOD'S PLAN FOR YOU

As I stated at the beginning of this book, God's plan for your life is only good—filled with peace, prosperity, health, and uplifting relationships. But to experience His plan, you need energy and strength.

Start getting energized daily by reading God's Word and praying. Let your desire echo the words of King David: "My life is an example to many, because you have been my strength and protection" (Ps. 71:7).

Claim the promise of God's strength and protection throughout your days. Read the scriptures in this book and memorize them, confessing them aloud at least once a day. Use them as spiritual medicine for your soul. Pray the Bible Cure prayers as you connect to God's power and energy for your life.

A **BIBLE CURE** Prayer for You

When I think of the wisdom and scope of God's plan, I fall to my knees and pray to the Father, the Creator of everything in heaven and on Earth. I pray that from His glorious, unlimited resources He will give me mighty inner strength through His Holy Spirit. And I pray that Christ will reveal the healing power of His Word to me as I trust in Him. May my roots go down deep into the soil of God's marvelous love. And may I have the power to understand, as all God's people should, how wide, how long, how high, and how deep His love for me really is. May I experience the revelation of the love of Christ,because faith works through love. Then I will be filled with the fullness of life and power that comes from God. Now glory be to God! By His mighty

*power at work within me, He is able to accomplish infinitely
more than I would ever dare to ask or hope. Amen.*

—Adapted from Ephesians 3:14–20

A **BIBLE CURE** Prescription

Trust God daily to renew your strength and energize you as you pray and read His Word. Review the self-test and symptom lists in this chapter, and quickly jot down any symptoms of chronic fatigue or fibromyalgia that you've been experiencing:

_____

_____

_____

_____

Write a prayer asking for God's help in applying the knowledge and wisdom you will learn in this book to energize you in overcoming these symptoms of fatigue:

_____

_____

_____

_____

Chapter 2

UNCOVERING THE CAUSES OF AND CONTRIBUTORS TO CHRONIC FATIGUE AND FIBROMYALGIA

T HE NUMBER ONE complaint that I hear from my patients is "I'm tired." My job is then to find out the underlying issue that's causing their loss of energy. Although fatigue has been discussed in medical literature for hundreds of years, determining its extent in people and its possible causes is something we've only recently begun to do. Fatigue can be complex and may be due to many medical problems, including anemia, low thyroid, medication side effects, diseases such as heart disease, depression, autoimmune disease, anxiety, lack of sleep, stress, poor diet, fatty liver, viral illnesses such as Epstein-Barr virus (EBV) and hepatitis C, chronic bacterial infections such as chronic sinusitis, and so on. Before I discuss the causes of fatigue I most commonly find among my patients, it's important for you to understand how your body produces energy in the first place.

FATIGUE AT THE CELLULAR LEVEL

The link between chronic fatigue and the cell's ability to produce energy is being studied more extensively now than it was when I first released this book in 2000. Let me explain how this connection between fatigue and mitochondrial function works.

Every cell in your body contains mitochondria, which are similar to little energy factories that convert nutrients into energy (ATP) by burning calories. That energy enables your cells to carry out their many functions in your body. But if you have mitochondrial dysfunction, inadequate energy is produced, and it's very difficult to overcome fatigue. Researchers found that the muscle tissue of a ninety-year-old man contained 95 percent damaged or dysfunctional mitochondria compared to practically no damage in a five-year-old child.[1]

Damage to mitochondria occurs naturally with aging, mainly as a result of accumulating oxidative stress from free radicals. However, many conditions, including infections, poor diet, chronic inflammation, chronic long-term stress, and heavy metal toxicity, can interfere with your body's ability to suppress oxidative damage. This sets the stage for mitochondrial dysfunction, leading to a lack of energy. Let's take a look at how various factors can contribute to chronic fatigue and fibromyalgia.

A BIBLE CURE Health Fact

- The heart muscle has thousands of mitochondria (mitochondria occupy 85 percent of the heart muscle's cell volume). You can see why the heart's cells have need of so much energy when you realize the heart never stops pumping, even during sleep.

- Skeletal muscles also have anywhere from hundreds to a couple thousand mitochondria, while fat cells have only a very few mitochondria.

SEVEN COMMON CAUSES OF OR CONTRIBUTORS TO CHRONIC FATIGUE

When the conditions mentioned above begin to affect a person's mitochondria, they take their toll on an individual's immune system, and chronic fatigue syndrome and fibromyalgia can result. Doctors commonly find a suppressed immune system and low adrenal function in their CFS patients. Let's take a closer look at the various causes of CFS and fibromyalgia.

1. Sleep disturbances

The most common cause of fatigue is simply lack of sleep—whether it's a result of inadequate sleep or poor quality of sleep. An estimated forty million Americans suffer from insomnia and other sleep disorders. Approximately 60 percent of American adults suffer from insomnia at least a few times each week. More than half the population will experience daytime drowsiness (fatigue).[2] Insomnia and not coping with stress are the most common causes of fatigue that I see in my practice.

Normal sleep actually occurs in cycles, with the average person experiencing about five or six sleep cycles during a normal night's sleep. Each sleep cycle typically lasts about sixty to ninety minutes. The first part of the cycle is composed of four stages. The deeper stages, stages three and four, are the most restful part of sleep. Stages one and two are more superficial sleep.

The second part of the cycle is the rapid eye movement, or the REM phase of sleep. During this phase of sleep, dreaming occurs. The majority of the time in the first ninety-minute cycle is spent in the first phase of the cycle, including the four stages, and only minutes are spent in the second phase of the REM cycle.

However, with each successive ninety-minute sleep cycle, less time is spent in phase one and more time is spent in phase two. In the final ninety-minute sleep cycle, before awakening in the morning, REM sleep takes up the majority of the time of the cycle, and only a few minutes are spent in phase one. Thus, many times before awakening, a lot people can remember their dreams.

Those who awaken during the transition from phase one to REM sleep are often very tired when they awaken in the morning, and thus they are very fatigued throughout the day. A variety of sleep disorders, which we will discuss in greater depth in chapter 5, can interrupt sleep and eventually trigger a pattern of chronic fatigue. Refer to *The New Bible Cure for Sleep Disorders* to learn more. Adequate amounts of refreshing sleep are very important in overcoming both chronic fatigue and fibromyalgia, and I will address the ways to get proper rest and refreshing sleep in chapter 5.

> But those who trust in the LORD will find new strength. They will soar high on wings like eagles. They will run and not grow weary. They will walk and not faint.
> —ISAIAH 40:31

2. Adrenal fatigue

Another major cause of fatigue is simply not coping with stress or excessive long-term stress, which eventually leads to adrenal fatigue. Adrenal fatigue is simply low adrenal function. Addison's disease is chronic adrenal failure where the adrenal glands do not function at all. If you keep the headlights of your car on all night, the battery will run down. At first you will be able to restart the car by jump-starting it. But if you leave the lights on continually night after night, eventually the battery will be so depleted that jump-starting it won't help.

A similar thing occurs in our bodies with excessive stress. We stress our bodies with our fast-paced lifestyles, juggling demanding jobs with even more demanding family responsibilities. Daily we dodge traffic jams, race to prepare dinner, and jog through malls and grocery stores to shop. Our schedules can leave us overworked, overwhelmed, spent, and exhausted.

As a family practitioner, I hear most of my regular patients complain of too much stress. Stress that persists for years and decades will eventually drain the adrenal glands and leave us tired, run-down, and chronically fatigued.

> So don't worry about these things, saying, "What will we eat? What will we drink? What will we wear?" These things dominate the thoughts of unbelievers, but your heavenly Father already knows all your needs. Seek the Kingdom of God above all else, and live righteously, and he will give you everything you need.
>
> —MATTHEW 6:31–33

Hans Selye is considered by many to be the "father of stress" since he was the first to document research related to the prolonged release of fight-or-flight hormones into the body and eventually to identify three stages of stress. Similar to Selye's stress classifications are three stages of adrenal fatigue. I discuss them in more detail in my book *Stress Less*, but I'd like to summarize them for you here.

Stage 1

In this stage of adrenal fatigue, long-term stress has caused the body to produce high levels of cortisol for a long period of time, usually accompanied by a prolonged decrease in DHEA and ongoing release of ACTH from the pituitary. The adrenals can eventually experience difficulty in meeting the demand for increased cortisol production placed upon them. When this happens, the body looks for other ways to facilitate cortisol production and will actually rob pregnenolone from the DHEA/sex hormone pathway to the progesterone/cortisol pathway to compensate. Total cortisol levels are elevated in Stage 1.

Stage 2

This transitional stage of adrenal fatigue signifies a continuing decline in cortisol levels, although ACTH stimulation remains high or even increases. There is a gradual change from increased to decreased stimulation. I've found that patients in this stage of adrenal fatigue may have low cortisol values in the morning, noon, or afternoon, but their nighttime cortisol levels are usually normal. This pattern of cortisol output is a marker of midstage adrenal exhaustion. DHEA is usually low or borderline low in this stage.

Stage 3

This final stage of adrenal fatigue is marked by the failure of the adrenals to produce enough cortisol to reach normal levels. Usually, DHEA levels are also low. The result is a hypothalamic-pituitary-adrenal axis "crash," in which nighttime cortisol levels also drop. There are usually severe imbalances in other hormone systems.

The body responds to emotional and mental stress as it would to a physical crisis. When you are faced with sudden danger, the alarm reaction phase of stress kicks in. The adrenal medulla releases adrenaline for extra strength and energy. In other words, your fight-or-flight response empowers you to either fight the battle or flee.

A **Bible Cure** *Health Fact*
Adrenal Glands

The adrenal glands are two very small glands, each about the size of a large grape, that sit on top of the kidneys. The main purpose of these glands is to give our bodies the stamina to cope with stress.

The adrenal gland has two parts. The inner part, called the medulla, mediates the "fight-or-flight" response. It secretes epinephrine and norepinephrine when an alarm reaction occurs. As a result, our blood pressure, heart rate, and respiratory rate all increase, and the body is prepared to "run" or "fight."

The outer shell is called the cortex and makes up about 80 percent of the gland. The adrenal cortex produces many different hormones, but they generally fall into three categories: glucocorticoids (most importantly cortisol), androgens (male hormones), and mineralocorticoids (primarily aldosterone).

For instance, if you were backpacking in the wilderness and stumbled upon a grizzly bear, you probably would not stand and fight the bear. Most likely you would flee. Adrenaline would shoot through your body, giving you nearly superhuman energy to help you escape from the bear.

With extreme stress, our bodies pump out potent chemicals that get us ready for fight or flight. But in modern society, we face emotional and mental stress every day, and these high-energy chemicals needed for fight or flight are still being released into our bodies during these stresses. In addition, when we are sitting in our boss's office or in traffic, we can neither fight nor flee. Nevertheless, these chemicals are still released, but fighting or fleeing actually lowers the levels of these stress chemicals in our bodies.

When the stress response is continually being set off in our bodies throughout the day for low-energy needs, we can end up stewing in our own juices (adrenaline and cortisol). Eventually we will become physically and emotionally burned out (the exhaustion stage). By our stress response triggering the release of adrenaline on low-energy needs, figuratively speaking our batteries eventually will become depleted—just like the car with its lights left on. This is also known as adrenal fatigue, in which the adrenals no longer produce enough cortisol to reach normal levels, lowering DHEA levels and creating severe imbalances in other hormone systems.

God designed this hormonal emergency alarm system to save our lives. But what happens if a person activates this system too many times for too many reasons? The alarm system actually becomes something harmful to the body, setting the stage for chronic illness such as CFS and fibromyalgia.

> You will keep in perfect peace all who trust in you, all whose thoughts are fixed on you! Trust in the LORD always, for the LORD GOD is the eternal Rock.
> —ISAIAH 26:3–4

3. Chronic infections

Another cause of chronic fatigue is chronic infections. People with CFS often have different and unusual infections at the same time, possibly linked to changes in the immune system of a person with CFS. With chronic fatigue, people usually have chronic, low-grade levels of infection. The most important infections fall within four categories:

1. Viral infections (Epstein-Barr virus, cytomegalovirus, human herpesvirus 6, viral hepatitis—these viruses can remain latent in your body long after the infection occurred, and they can reactivate during CFS). People with CFS are often referred to an infectious disease specialist when EBV (Epstein-Barr virus) infection is the precipitating event that has triggered the chronic fatigue.

2. Yeast infections (candidiasis). I will explain more about this below.

3. Parasitic infections

4. Bacterial infections (chronic sinusitis, chronic bronchitis, chronic prostatitis, mycoplasmal infections, Chlamydia, Lyme disease, and periodontal disease) are commonly associated with chronic fatigue. Upper respiratory and sinus infections are the most common among CFS patients. The link between sinus infection and chronic fatigue has become so well documented that 200,000 sinus surgeries a year are now performed in order to alleviate the fatigue that accompanies this condition.[3]

Patients with CFS and fibromyalgia need to be checked for Lyme disease. I usually perform the Igenex Lyme disease test (see Appendix B). I also check for chronic viral infections including EBV, CMV, and HHV6, as well as viral hepatitis. I also find a strong link to chronic sinus infections, so I often check a CT scan of the sinuses to rule out a chronic sinus infection. I usually treat these infections with herbs, homeopathics, IV nutrients, and on occasion antibiotics. However, I commonly find that when I address the other causes and contributors of CFS and fibromyalgia, the immune system is usually recharged and begins to properly fight off infections. This is why I also place all my patients on vitamin D3 and optimize their vitamin D3 blood level to 50–100 ng/ml, which usually improves immune function.

Since candidiasis (chronic yeast infection) is one of the most common infections causing chronic fatigue that I see in my practice, I'd like to discuss it here.

Candidiasis

Candida albicans is a yeast organism that has been around for thousands of years. This yeast is normally present in the gastrointestinal tracts of healthy people. Yeast is a single-celled organism that thrives on the surface of other living things, including our fruits, grains, vegetables, and even our skin. Yeast is similar to fungus. Mushrooms, molds, and mildew are all different types of yeast.

Candida yeast normally lives in the gastrointestinal tract and the vagina. It coexists harmoniously among trillions of bacteria. Many of these good bacteria (called the lactobacillus) prevent the overgrowth of yeast, prevent buildup of disease-forming bacteria, and even synthesize certain vitamins.

Only relatively small numbers of yeast candida are normally present in our gastrointestinal tracts. The beneficial bacteria balance the yeast so that they are unable to grow out of control. Our immune systems also help to keep the yeast in check. However, when we take potent antibiotics, especially over a prolonged period of time, much of the good bacteria are destroyed, and the critical balance of microorganisms in the gastrointestinal tract is upset. When too many of the lactobacilli and other beneficial bacteria have been killed, the yeast can grow unimpeded.

Other factors that can cause yeast overgrowth include cortisone, birth control pills, pregnancy, environmental chemicals, diabetes, certain foods (especially sugars), and allergies. Allergies and viral infections tend to drain the immune system. When the immune system is weakened, yeast is able to multiply unchecked. Deficiencies in digestive secretions can also lead to an overgrowth of candida. Pancreatic enzymes, hydrochloric acid, and bile will help prevent the overgrowth of candida.

Candidiasis can cause chronic nasal congestion or chronic sinusitis; impaired memory; distractibility; irritability and agitation; inability to concentrate; feeling drunk without consuming alcohol; craving for sugar; anxiety; depression; troublesome vaginal burning, itching, or discharge; fatigue; and insomnia. Gastrointestinal symptoms include bloating, swelling, spastic colon, IBS, diarrhea and/or constipation, loud intestinal rumblings, cramping, excessive gas, itching of the anus, mucus in the stools, food sensitivity or intolerance, and heartburn.

While these are the most common symptoms of candidiasis that I see, candidiasis can also affect nearly every system of the body, including the immune system, endocrine system, and genitourinary system.

I see cases of candidiasis on a daily basis in my practice, and I believe most of it is caused by the overuse of antibiotics by physicians to treat acne and chronic or recurrent infections such as sinusitis, bronchitis, and prostatitis. Decades ago, when antibiotics were first used, they could kill almost any form of bacteria. However, bacteria have changed their genetic makeup and have become increasingly resistant to the antibiotics. Now, resistant bacteria have become stronger and stronger, so that some strands of bacteria may be resistant to almost all forms of antibiotics.

While I am not against the use of antibiotics, for they have saved countless lives, I do believe they should be used sparingly. Many physicians prescribe them for flu and colds, although we know that antibiotics do not kill viruses. Some patients believe that antibiotics are good for all infections and often pressure their physicians to prescribe them. The extended use of antibiotics for treating acne, chronic sinus infections, and chronic prostate infections will likely create another disease that very few people and even physicians are aware of: chronic candidiasis!

Excessive yeast overgrowth will actually compete with the body for nutrition and rob it of many nutrients. It releases toxic by-products such as alcohol, acetaldehyde, and as many as seventy-nine different toxins that can circulate through the bloodstream and affect other organs and tissues. This places a tremendous burden on the immune system. A vicious cycle of continual and progressive draining of the immune system begins. I've written an entire Bible Cure book on candida and yeast infections and encourage you to refer to it if you need more information.

In addition, the inflammation in the gastrointestinal tract caused by yeast infections creates a "leaky gut" in which food proteins and other foreign substances are able to travel directly into the circulatory system, often triggering food allergies and food sensitivities in our bodies. This is one of the reasons why so many patients with chronic candidiasis develop severe food sensitivities and allergies as well as food intolerances. This cycle causes additional fatigue, and thus the cycle continues.

4. Hypothyroidism and hormone imbalance

Hypothyroidism. Think of your thyroid gland as similar to your body's gas pedal. It regulates your body's metabolic rate. If your thyroid is underactive, you typically can gain weight, become intolerant to cold temperatures, and experience achiness, confusion, constipation, and fatigue. Your thyroid produces two primary hormones: thyroxine (T4) and triiodothyronine (T3). When you have CFS, your body may not be able to adequately convert T4 into T3. After seeing hundreds of people in my practice struggle to convert T4 to T3, I have identified the following main reasons for their poor conversion:

- Chronic unremitting stress
- Adrenal fatigue
- Medications that interfere with conversion
- Consumption of certain foods, such as soy, or excessive alcohol
- Excessive consumption of raw cruciferous vegetables (this is rare)
- Low-fat, low-carbohydrate, or low-protein diets

Other common causes of low thyroid function in chronic fatigue and fibromyalgia patients include Hashimoto's thyroiditis, an autoimmune condition; dysfunction of the hypothalamus; and thyroid receptor resistance, in which it takes higher doses of T3 hormone since the thyroid receptors are resistant.

Low sex hormone levels are also associated with CFS/fibromyalgia. This can affect both men and women. Treating low testosterone levels in men can lead to dramatic improvements in energy levels and overall sense of well-being among those suffering from CFS and fibromyalgia.

In women, deficiencies of progesterone and testosterone can exacerbate symptoms of chronic fatigue. Progesterone is usually the first hormone that becomes deficient in women with CFS and fibromyalgia. However, restoring balance by using bioidentical progesterone usually helps improve sleep, calms the emotions, helps balance the adrenal glands, and improves symptoms of CFS and fibromyalgia.

Estrogen deficiencies can play a major role in women with CFS and fibromyalgia. It's no secret that low estrogen levels are associated with fatigue, brain fog, PMS, low serotonin, poor sleep, poor libido, and other problems. Hormonal imbalances are commonly associated with menopause but can occur at any time in a woman's life.

For years I have been recommending bioidentical hormone therapy for my female patients who suffer from low hormone levels. Unfortunately, most physicians use the synthetic forms of hormones. I encourage you to talk to your doctor or find a physician trained in bioidentical hormone replacement about hormone therapy options. If your doctor is not open to the idea of bioidentical hormone replacement therapy, get a second opinion. (See Appendix B for help in finding a board-certified doctor who is knowledgeable in bioidentical hormone therapy.)

A BIBLE CURE *Health Fact*

Oxytocin Deficiency: Contributing Factions, Symptoms, and Associated Conditions

The following lists outline signs of oxytocin deficiency, factors that contribute to lower levels of oxytocin, and conditions that are associated with low levels of oxytocin.

Signs of oxytocin deficiency

- Pale skin
- Tense body and muscles

- Serious expressions, forced smiles, tense facial muscles
- Stressed or unhappy look in the eyes
- Tiny wrinkles in the face
- Painful tender points (fibromyalgia)
- Asocial tendencies, poor relationship skills
- Irritability or depression

Factors that contribute to low levels of oxytocin

- Drinking excessive fluids/water
- Loneliness or detachment, as displayed by a lack of family connections and social contacts
- Bad social experiences
- Chronic stressful situations
- Prolonged negative emotions such as fear or anger
- Drug abuse

Conditions associated with low oxytocin

- Fibromyalgia
- Anxiety disorders
- Depression
- Hormone imbalances
- Prader-Willi syndrome
- Parkinson's disease
- Multiple sclerosis
- AIDS
- Autism
- Schizophrenia

Oxytocin, an important hormone and neurotransmitter in the brain, is often low in people with fibromyalgia. The lower a person's oxytocin level, the more sensitive they are to stress and the harder it is for them to deal with or manage their stress. Some research indicates that people who have had stressful or traumatic things happen during childhood have the lowest oxytocin levels, and their oxytocin levels appear to be "stuck," remaining low their entire lives.

More research is needed before oxytocin becomes an accepted treatment for fibromyalgia, but the results of research thus far look promising. Injections have been found to cause deep muscle relaxation for several hours, creating a feeling of being in a pleasant relaxed state with no anxiety or tenseness. Oxytocin also comes in a sublingual form and a nose spray.

People who are pale and have cold hands and feet seem to receive the greatest benefit from oxytocin treatments, experiencing decreased pain, increased energy, and mental clarity. Others who have been injected with oxytocin report experiencing:

- The ability to cope with stress and solve stressful problems with less anxiety
- The ability to appease conflicts with people more easily
- The perception that other people are kinder and full of good intentions
- The perception that the atmosphere of various situations is more positive

It's likely that chronic stress depletes oxytocin stores. A deficit in oxytocin not only robs a person of its pain-killing effects but also sets them up to develop a pain sensation all over the body—a phenomenon often experienced by people with severe fibromyalgia.

A BIBLE CURE *Health Tip*
Curly Compact Fluorescent Light Bulbs Contain Mercury

Those new (curly) compact fluorescent lights (CFLs) are replacing the traditional round incandescent bulbs. CFLs are safe as long as the bulbs don't break. If the bulbs are cracked, broken, or not disposed of properly, the mercury vapors that are released into the air can pose a health hazard. According to a recent report on FOX News, there is enough mercury in one fluorescent light bulb to contaminate six thousand gallons of water.

If a CFL bulb breaks, the EPA suggests the following steps:

- People and pets must leave the room immediately.
- Open a window or door and air the room for five to ten minutes.
- Turn off central air or heating system.
- Collect all broken glass and visible powder using wet cloths; never use a vacuum or broom.
- Do not leave the bulb fragments or cleanup materials indoors. Put all debris and cleanup materials in sealable containers and leave them in an outdoor trash can or protected area until they can be disposed of properly.
- If possible, allow the room to continue to air via open window or door for several hours.[4]

5. Heavy metal toxicity

Another cause of chronic fatigue is heavy metal toxicity. Heavy metals that accumulate in the body and cause toxicity include lead, cadmium, aluminum, and arsenic. However, the most common heavy metal toxicity is mercury toxicity. People are most commonly exposed to mercury through contaminated fish, silver amalgam fillings, and immunizations with thimerosal (a mercury preservative). The word *amalgam* literally means "mixed with mercury," and amalgam fillings are exactly that: they are 52 percent mercury mixed with a combination of copper, zinc, tin, and silver.[5]

In the past century the amount of environmental mercury has increased thirtyfold, with 70 percent of the new sources of mercury being manmade. Sources of mercury in the environment include:

- Metal mining and smelting
- Municipal waste incineration
- Sewage and medical waste incineration
- Coal-fired industrial plants and chlor-alkali plants that use mercury to make the chlorine used in plastics, pesticides, and PVC pipes
- Cement manufacturing
- Electrical products, fluorescent lamps, thermometers, thermostats, and electrical switches (this category is the largest use of mercury)
- Disposal of mercury-containing products in landfills and mercury spills that occur when mercury-containing products are broken
- Fish that contain mercury (see the Bible Cure Health Fact titled "Watch for Mercury in Fish")

Symptoms of mercury toxicity (many doctors dismiss these symptoms or blame them on aging) include fatigue and listlessness; impairment of peripheral vision; a "pins and needles" feeling, usually in the hands, feet, and around the mouth; lack of coordination; impairment of speech, hearing, and walking; tremors; insomnia and changes in sleeping patterns; neuromuscular changes (weakness, muscle atrophy, twitching); headaches; emotional changes (mood swings, irritability, nervousness, excessive shyness, lack of motivation, hopelessness); changes in nerve responses; deficits in cognitive function (brain fog and confusion); skin rashes and dermatitis; memory loss; and mental disturbances.

A **BIBLE CURE** Health Fact

Watch for Mercury in Fish

The following is a list of fish and their reported mercury levels. As you can see, salmon is very low in mercury.

- Tilefish, 3 oz. (golden bass or golden snapper), 1.45 ppm
- Shark, 3 oz., 0.99 ppm
- Swordfish, 3 oz., 0.97 ppm
- King mackerel, 3 oz., 0.73 ppm
- Canned tuna (light), 3 oz., 0.12 ppm
- Cod, 3 oz., 0.09 ppm
- Crabs, 3 oz., 0.06 ppm
- Flounder or sole, 3 oz., 0.05 ppm
- Scallops, 3 oz., 0.05 ppm
- Catfish, 3 oz., 0.05 ppm
- Salmon, 3 oz., 0.01 ppm[7]

Mercury poisoning has possible links with multiple sclerosis, Parkinson's disease, Alzheimer's disease, autoimmune diseases, pregnancy complications, infertility, cancer, leukemia, depression, and chronic fatigue.[6] See chapter 1 of my book *What You Don't Know May Be Killing You* for my specific recommendations for detoxing your body if you suspect you are dealing with mercury poisoning.

6. Food allergies and sensitivities

Over the years I have found that chronic fatigue and fibromyalgia symptoms can also be triggered by food allergies, delayed food sensitivities, and excessive intake of sugars and high glycemic carbohydrates. Remember when you ate a big plate of pasta for lunch or pancakes for breakfast and felt sleepy shortly thereafter? This is a direct result of the effect these foods have on your body's serotonin levels.

Delayed food sensitivities can also cause fatigue after meals (wheat, dairy, corn, soy, nightshades, eggs, tree nuts, and peanuts are common causes of delayed food sensitivities), but the symptoms can be delayed for several hours to several days, making them much harder to detect.

Food allergies and sensitivities can also cause adrenal stress. Therefore I suggest a comprehensive food allergy or food sensitivity test in order to determine the foods to which you are allergic or sensitive. (See Appendix B.)

If you have food allergies or sensitivities, I first recommend that you avoid all foods that you are sensitive to for six weeks. Also rotate your foods by eating different foods each day for four days and then start the rotation over. For example, if you are sensitive to dairy, corn, tomatoes, and pork, eliminate these foods for six weeks and then rotate them back into your diet every four days. If you continue to have symptoms, then avoid that food altogether.

Some of my patients are so sensitive that they need to rotate all their foods daily. For example (assuming they are not sensitive to these foods), they might be able to have turkey, green beans, brown rice, and apples for one day. But the next day they need to avoid these foods and instead choose chicken, cabbage, asparagus, lentils, and pears. Then on day three they need to choose lean organic beef or steak, broccoli, sweet potatoes, and blueberries. Day four's choices might be wild salmon or tongol tuna along with different veggies, starches, and fruits. Then they can start over and eat turkey and the other foods from day one again. This might sound like a strict program, but it has helped many of my patients with severe food allergies and sensitivities to get their life back again. See Appendix B for more information on food sensitivity testing.

In addition to rotating your foods, I recommend that you decrease or eliminate from your diet all processed starches such as white bread, white flour, white rice, sugar, pastries, packaged foods, and potato chips. Increase your intake of vegetables, lean meats, brown rice, millet bread, and good fats such as flaxseed oil, extra-virgin olive oil, almonds, walnuts, and fish oil. Drink at least 2–3 quarts of alkaline water a day and follow my candida diet in *The Bible Cure for Candida and Yeast Infections.*

I also believe that an important technique to help you "desensitize" from these foods (to help your body to no longer be sensitive to them) is NAET, which is a form of allergy desensitization using acupressure. I have seen hundreds of patients desensitized from food allergies and sensitivities by using this technique.

A **BIBLE CURE** *Health Tip*
The Coca Pulse Test

Perform the Coca Pulse Test. Take your pulse for one minute prior to eating. Then place a bite of the food to which you might be allergic on your tongue. After thirty seconds, recheck your pulse. If the pulse rate increases by more than six beats per minute, you may be sensitive or allergic to the food. The higher the pulse goes up, usually the more severe the allergy or sensitivity.

7. Neurotransmitter imbalance

To understand how neurotransmitter imbalance affects chronic fatigue and fibromyalgia sufferers, you must begin with a basic knowledge of what certain neurotransmitters do. Three key neurotransmitters related to how we experience and handle stress are norepinephrine, serotonin, and dopamine.

During the fight-or-flight stress response, norepinephrine and its sister hormone epinephrine (better known as adrenaline) cause an increase of blood to the brain that makes a person more focused and alert during a crisis. When our norepinephrine levels are low, we can feel sluggish, tired, or exhausted, and often have trouble concentrating on one thing. This often propels an out-of-control eating lifestyle.

Serotonin is the neurotransmitter responsible for giving you the sense of being happy, full, and satisfied. An imbalance of this neurotransmitter is associated with problems sleeping, cravings for sweets (especially chocolate) and carbohydrates, binge eating, panic attacks, compulsive eating, mental fixation on food, and obsessive-compulsive disorder (OCD).

Dopamine is the "pleasure neurotransmitter," enabling you to both feel and seek out pleasure. When your dopamine levels are consistently low, you become prone to developing any kind of addiction—drugs, alcohol, cigarettes, gambling, shopping, sex, etc. Like the other two deficiencies, an imbalance of dopamine can make you prone to depression, irritability, or moodiness.

Chronic stress can cause deficiencies in all three of these neurotransmitters, which can lead to depression and a whole host of symptoms and contribute to chronic illnesses such as fibromyalgia and chronic fatigue. For more information on neurotransmitter imbalance, please see my book *The New Bible Cure for Depression and Anxiety.*

YOUR FATIGUE

You've probably realized by now that chronic fatigue is not a simple disease. Many factors, or a combination of factors, may be responsible for your fatigue. As we have discussed some major causes of or contributors to chronic fatigue and fibromyalgia, have you seen your own symptoms? Throughout the rest of this book I will be providing natural and spiritual remedies that will arm you to battle your enemy and defeat chronic fatigue and fibromyalgia and their symptoms forever!

A **BIBLE CURE** *Prayer for You*

Lord Jesus, thank You for beginning the process of total restoration in my body. Your power and wisdom are greater than every symptom and every disease. Give me divinely ordained grace to undergo a special time of self-examination as I seek to discover the causes of chronic fatigue or fibromyalgia in my life. Help me to develop lifestyle changes that will set me free from these illnesses for the rest of my days. In Jesus's name, amen.

A **BIBLE CURE** Prescription

Write down any symptoms of CFS or fibromyalgia that you experience on a chronic basis.

_____

_____

_____

Which causes of CFS or fibromyalgia do you feel apply to your life?

_____

_____

_____

Chapter 3

REFUEL WITH NUTRITION

Y OUR PLAN TO overcome CFS and fibromyalgia begins with good nutrition. You wouldn't put water into your gas tank and expect your car to run, would you? Your car needs to be fueled properly, according to its design. Well, the designer of your body, God, has provided just the right fuel for you!

> Then God said, "Look! I have given you every seed-bearing plant throughout the earth and all the fruit trees for your food. And I have given every green plant as food for all the wild animals, the birds in the sky, and the small animals that scurry along the ground— everything that has life." And that is what happened. Then God looked over all he had made, and he saw that it was very good!
>
> —GENESIS 1:29–31

As a foundation in overcoming CFS and fibromyalgia and being energized to enjoy life, I strongly recommend that you follow the eating plan found in my book *Dr. Colbert's "I Can Do This" Diet*. The carefully calculated protein-carb-fat ratio of this eating plan will benefit you greatly, no matter the cause of your fatigue. If your diet contains excessive sugar, fat, starch, and salt, you are probably experiencing fatigue and even chronic fatigue. Balanced nutrition helps your body fight off fatigue and sustains you through demanding and stressful situations.

INSURING PROPER DIGESTION

Since the original printing of this book, a new development has become increasingly important in the discussion of chronic fatigue: hypochlorhydria. A person with hypochlorhydria does not produce adequate amounts of stomach acid (hydrochloric acid) and therefore does not adequately digest food and absorb its nutrients. This leaves cells weak from undernourishment and puts a person at increased risk of food poisoning, *H. Pylori* bacterial infection, and parasites because this acid is responsible for killing pathogenic bacteria and parasites that enter the body via food.

Low stomach acid plays a significant role in CFS, fibromyalgia, and brain fog;[1] it is also linked to various diseases and disorders, including:

- Acne rosacea
- Allergies
- Asthma
- Autoimmune diseases
- Celiac disease
- Chronic hepatitis
- Diabetes mellitus
- Dry skin
- Eczema
- Gallbladder disease
- Hypoglycemia

- Lupus
- Macular degeneration
- Multiple chemical sensitivity
- Pernicious anemia
- Poor night vision
- Psoriasis
- Reflux (GERD)
- Rheumatic arthritis
- Stomach ulcers/helicobacter pylori
- Thyroid disorders
- Urticaria (hives)
- Vitiligo
- Weak adrenals
- Weak nails

Insufficient stomach acid may allow proteins to pass through the intestines undigested, and carbohydrates are left to ferment. Low stomach acid also causes malabsorption of minerals like zinc, manganese, and calcium.

Hypochlorhydria can be caused by a number of things: B vitamin deficiency, consuming excess carbs, hypothyroidism, food sensitivities, infection, soda consumption, and aging. But the most common cause is stress. Symptoms of low stomach acid include belching or gas within an hour of eating, bloating and stomach pain shortly after eating, bad breath, loss of taste for meat or trouble digesting it, reflux or heartburn, nausea after taking supplements, brittle fingernails, undigested food in stool, constipation, poor appetite or feeling overly full easily, multiple food sensitivities, low iron levels, estrogen buildup, acne rosacea, depression, and fatigue.

If you experience any of these symptoms, talk to your doctor about having a Heidelberg test or a trial on a hydrochloric acid supplement. (See Appendix B.)

OVERCOMING CANDIDIASIS

If your CFS or fibromyalgia symptoms are caused by candidiasis or food allergies, a specialized diet for three to six months usually will change your life completely.

Symptoms of candidiasis include fatigue, mental cloudiness, disorientation, confusion, insomnia, mood swings, irritability, headaches, anxiety, depression, memory loss, hyperactivity, and attention-deficit disorder. For a complete self-examination to determine if a yeast infection is the hidden source of symptoms you've been experiencing, please see my book *The Bible Cure for Candida and Yeast Infections*.

Cookies, candies, cakes, pies, and soft drinks will feed candida to the point at which the yeast grows out of control. Changing your diet is the most important thing you can do to begin treating chronic candidiasis. Start by avoiding, eliminating, or radically reducing the following:

1. *All sweets.* Sweets include white sugar (sucrose, fructose, glucose, galactose, and sorbitol) and all other sugars, including corn syrup, dextrose, barley malt, honey, molasses, brown rice syrup, and even fruit juice. Avoid all pastries, breads, and other bakery goods.

2. *Milk products.* Milk and all milk products should be restricted. The sugar in milk, which is lactose, actually feeds the yeast, as does regular sugar. Cheeses especially should be avoided because they contain yeast or mold, and blue cheese, or Roquefort, is one of the worst. You should also avoid fermented dairy products such as yogurt, buttermilk, and sour cream.

3. *Vinegar.* Foods containing vinegar, such as soy sauce, barbecue sauce, steak sauce, mustard, ketchup, mayonnaise, salad dressings, horseradish, and pickled vegetables, should be avoided by many with candida.

   (Note: If you cannot limit or avoid yeast- and mold-containing foods, you should at least avoid sugary foods and beverages such as cakes, pies, candy, colas, juices, and pastries.)

4. *Meats that have been processed or smoked should also be avoided.* These include bacon, sausage, ham, smoked turkey, and other processed meats.

5. *Dried fruits,* including raisins, figs, and dates, should also be avoided.

6. *Coffee* is OK as long as you use no cream or sugar.

7. *Peanuts and peanut butter* should be avoided since they commonly contain mold.

8. *Melons.* Limit or avoid most melons, especially cantaloupe.

9. *All alcoholic beverages,* including beer, wine, and mixed drinks, should be avoided since they contain extremely high amounts of yeast along with simple carbohydrates that feed yeast.

10. *Foods that trigger allergies or sensitivities.* The next category of foods to avoid is foods that trigger allergies or sensitivities. Most people with candidiasis have many food sensitivities. The most common ones are eggs, dairy, wheat, soy, nuts, and corn. However, in order to determine which foods you are allergic or sensitive to, have a food sensitivity test such as the SAGE test. (See Appendix B.)

11. *High-glycemic carbohydrates.* Finally, it is best to limit your intake of high-glycemic carbohydrates, including potatoes (especially instant potatoes), white rice, popcorn, high-sugar cereals, chips, and most crackers. Some good grain alternatives are buckwheat, amaranth, quinoa, millet, and brown rice.

Try to avoid both yeast- and mold-containing foods as much as possible. However, yeast- and mold-containing foods such as breads, enriched flour, alcoholic beverages, vinegar, aged cheeses, fermented dairy products, mushrooms, peanut butter, and canned juices do not actually make candida grow. When people develop symptoms from eating yeast- or mold-containing foods, it's usually because they are allergic or sensitive to the yeast.

Leftovers may contain mold too. I'm sure that you've noticed how green mold grows on opened cheese that has been left sitting in the refrigerator for a few weeks.

But remember, the main foods that make yeast or candida grow are high-sugar foods! Sugar-containing foods are the main nutrients for yeast. These include not only simple sugars such as sucrose, fructose, corn syrup, honey, fruit juice, and maple syrup, but also even milk and dairy products (which contain milk sugar called lactose) and high-glycemic carbohydrates such as white rice and potatoes. All of these may contribute to excessive yeast overgrowth.

What Can I Eat?

To simplify things, I will list the following food groups that you may freely enjoy while you are on the candida diet.

Meat and fish proteins. These include chicken, turkey, lean beef (I prefer organic, free-range meat and pastured poultry), veal, wild game, lamb, ham, and pork. (Pork as well as ham are forbidden in the Book of Leviticus in the Bible, but if you must eat them, be sure they are very lean.) Also included in the list of protein foods are shellfish, including shrimp, lobster, crab, and so forth. (All varieties of shellfish are also forbidden in Leviticus under ancient Judaic law.) Wild salmon, sardines, tongol tuna, and most other fish are recommended as long as they are wild-caught and not farm-raised. Also, don't add breading to any meat or fish during cooking, and do not deep-fry.

Vegetables. Low-glycemic vegetables include broccoli, brussels sprouts, celery, cabbage, cauliflower, carrots, collard greens, and eggplant. Leafy greens include lettuce, spinach, parsley, collard greens, beet greens, watercress, kale, chard (mustard greens), onions, bell peppers, snow peas, string beans, tomatoes, turnips, eggplant, and artichokes.

Grains and nuts. These include amaranth, quinoa, millet, brown rice, wild rice, and buckwheat. Nuts and seeds include almonds, flaxseeds, sunflower seeds, pumpkin seeds, pecans, and Brazil nuts. Nuts are difficult for many people to digest. Therefore I recommend that you soak them in filtered or distilled water overnight for at least twelve hours, preferably in a glass container or jar. Drain the water and store the nuts in the refrigerator in an airtight container. This causes the nuts to sprout, which makes them easier to digest.

Oils. Organic, unrefined, expeller-pressed vegetable oils, organic butter, and organic extra-virgin olive oil are permitted. (Vegetable oils include sunflower oil, safflower oil, pumpkin seed oil, and flaxseed oil.) Use oils in salad dressings, and cook with organic butter, coconut oil, high-oleic, expeller-pressed safflower oil, or sunflower oil. Do not cook with flaxseed oil.

Margarine and all refined oils, such as most cooking oils found in grocery stores, should be eliminated from the diet. Margarine and refined oils can contribute to a variety of degenerative and inflammatory diseases.

Carbs. If you are sensitive to wheat products and if they cause you bloating, gas, or a lot of rumbling in your stomach, then I recommend that you avoid wheat bread, wheat crackers, pasta, pancakes, and waffles. Most of my patients with candida do not tolerate wheat well, but they do well with millet bread or brown rice bread or pasta.

LIVER DETOXIFICATION

Excessive yeast overgrowth is often linked with leaky gut (also called increased intestinal permeability) and too many poisonous toxins in the liver. If you are experiencing candida overgrowth, you may need to undergo a nutritional program to repair the GI tract and to detox your liver. Detoxifying the liver can be extremely important in overcoming severe candidiasis.

The most important way to detox the liver and repair the GI tract is to identify your delayed food sensitivities by a special blood test called the SAGE test. (See Appendix B.) If the basic candida diet is not relieving your symptoms of candida, then there is a very good chance that you have delayed food sensitivities, a leaky gut, and a toxic liver.

Let me explain. When a patient has severe candidiasis of the intestinal tract, the yeast transforms from the normal budding friendly form to the hyphael form. This form damages and inflames the lining of the small intestine by damaging the tight junctions between the mucosal cells. This in turn allows increased absorption of partially digested foods and proteins. With increased intestinal permeability, large food proteins, antigens, and toxins are absorbed into the body. The body may view these foods as foreign invaders and may form antibodies against them. IgG antibodies and immune complexes are formed, which may inflame and damage other tissues and organs, especially the liver. The food elimination and rotational diet helps to heal the GI tract, which helps to detox the liver. It is also important to kill the excessive yeast in the GI tract and restore the beneficial bacteria. I sometimes have patients take a glutathione-boosting supplement, milk thistle, lipoic acid, and selenium to restore normal liver function. (See Appendix B for specific product recommendations.)

SPEAKING FRANKLY ABOUT FIBER

Many individuals don't get enough fiber and water in their diets—and chronic constipation is the unpleasant result. In order to clear yeast from the GI (gastrointestinal) tract, it's important to have regular bowel movements—at least one every day. Enjoy lots of raw vegetables in your diet, and drink at least two quarts of water a day.

Fiber binds yeast and prevents it from being reabsorbed in the body. You may also consider taking a fiber supplement, such as freshly ground flaxseeds or a fiber supplement. (See Appendix B.) Psyllium fiber supplements are commonly sold over the counter;

however, I advise you to take one that does not contain sugar or NutraSweet.

THE GOOD GUYS

As I have already mentioned, getting rid of bad bacteria with antibiotics can cause the good bacteria, to be killed off too. Without the good bacteria, yeast usually grows out of control.

Trillions of these good bacteria live in our intestinal tract and keep the intestines healthy by feeding on the waste, fungus, yeast, and harmful bacteria. The good guys also produce vitamins, hormones, and proteins that our bodies need.

Therefore, during the process of clearing yeast from the body, you need to take in beneficial bacteria (probiotics) so that the bowel will be recolonized with them.

I recommend approximately 100 to 200 billion or more colony-forming units of beneficial bacteria. It's best to take them upon waking in the morning or on an empty stomach. (See "Supplements and Medications for Candidiasis" and Appendix B for specific probiotics I recommend.)

LIVESTOCK AND ANTIBIOTICS

Did you realize that much of the meat we eat every day is loaded with antibiotics? "Some 60 percent to 80 percent of all cattle, sheep, swine, and poultry in the United States will be given antibiotics at some point. In addition to treating specific diseases, much of the approximately 19 million pounds of antibiotics used annually in agriculture are added to feed or water to promote growth and to help prevent animals in close quarters from transmitting diseases. In these cases, antibiotics are administered in doses much lower than those required to treat specific infections. Using antibiotics in this 'subtherapeutic' way allows more animals to be raised at lower costs."[2]

Every time you eat a steak or a chicken thigh, you are probably ingesting antibiotics. These antibiotics are killing off the beneficial bacteria in our bodies and making us increasingly prone to getting candidiasis. It's critically important to take in good bacteria daily to replace what the antibiotics in the meat that we eat are destroying. Please refer to "Supplements and Medications for Candidiasis" for my probiotic program for patients with candida.

GET STARTED!

Since chronic fatigue and fibromyalgia may range from mild tiredness to extreme exhaustion to distressing muscle pain, it is best to seek nutritional treatment early. The longer it persists, the longer it usually takes to turn the problem around. Make a decision to start eating healthy foods and drinking healthy beverages now.

> Give all your worries and cares to God, for he cares about you.
>
> —1 PETER 5:7

CONCLUSION

Whether yeast overgrowth, food sensitivities or allergies, or any of the other culprits that may be taxing your immune system cause or contribute to your chronic fatigue and fibromyalgia and steal your energy, the first place to go for answers is always Jesus Christ. He understands your body, for He created it. And He loves and understands you. And just as every good father wants the best for his children, He longs for you to experience a richer, more abundant life.

Have you ever used sugar or breads and pastries to fill a physical or even an emotional void? Many Christians use sodas or other sugary foods and beverages as their comforter instead of the Holy Spirit, the true Comforter. Sugar is neither your comforter nor the source of your power or energy in life—God is. In fact, the Bible says that the bread of life is Jesus Himself. Your dependence on yeast products in the natural may be robbing you of a more important spiritual focus in your life—Jesus Christ, the bread of life.

If you have a dependence on bread and yeast or sugar products in your life, then turn to the true bread of life as your source. You must be willing to lay sugar on the altar for at least a season, usually three to six months, in order to overcome candidiasis. When you become hungry for bread or sugar products, remember His promise to you: "I am the bread of life. Whoever comes to me will never be hungry again. Whoever believes in me will never be thirsty" (John 6:35).

A **BIBLE CURE** Prayer for You

Lord Jesus, break any dependence I have on sugar and bread and fill my hunger for sugar and bread with Your living bread. Help me to discern how dependent I am on sugar and yeast products. Give me the strength and willpower to eliminate these products from my life and to feed on Your bread and drink Your living water. Amen.

A **BIBLE CURE** *Prescription*

What products do you need to eliminate from your diet?

_____

_____

_____

Describe how dependent you are on sugar. Then make a decision to lay sugar on the altar and allow the Holy Spirit to be your comforter, not sugar.

_____

_____

_____

List the healthy foods you will include in your diet:

_____

_____

_____

Write a prayer asking God to free you from any dependence you may have on sugar or yeast products.

_____

_____

_____

Chapter 4

RECHARGE WITH EXERCISE

P EOPLE WITH CFS and fibromyalgia usually hate to exercise since they are exhausted and often have painful trigger points throughout their bodies, causing very tender muscles. However, I can promise you that nothing is more invigorating than participating in a regular exercise routine.

The apostle Paul said, "I discipline my body like an athlete, training it to do what it should. Otherwise, I fear that after preaching to others I myself might be disqualified" (1 Cor. 9:27). Like the apostle Paul, I believe in the powerful benefits of exercise. Regular exercise can help to relieve both fatigue and muscle pain.

The exercises I mention in this chapter will help you to overcome the fatigue caused by excessive stress over a long period of time. I will begin with basic steps you can take to help overcome even the most severe fatigue and show you how to build upon this as your fatigue and pain become less severe.

THE IMPORTANCE OF RELAXATION

Since stress is a major contributor to CFS and fibromyalgia, I want to first address how to better manage your stress level through relaxation. You cannot live in this world without experiencing stress, but there are ways you can help to relieve the effects of stress upon your body. The goal here is not to tell you to eliminate stress but to help you learn how to manage the toll it takes on your body.

You may not have ever thought about your stress level in relationship to your chronic fatigue or fibromyalgia, but the muscle tension you may be experiencing with these two conditions are actually your body's way of informing you that you're under stress. Most people don't stop to notice they are developing tense muscles until that tension reaches the point where they have a full-blown headache, sore neck, sore shoulders, backache, TMJ, or pain in the thighs or the various tender trigger points known as fibromyalgia.

The good news is that no matter how much stress you may have accumulated and how it is expressed in your body, it is a scientific fact that nearly all people can use the same basic relaxation techniques with wonderful results. I want to introduce several practical techniques that are available and effective for enhanced relaxation. I will then lead you to build upon your muscle relaxation by adding stretching and less strenuous exercises.

Deep-Breathing Exercises

Deep breathing or abdominal breathing, which involves deep inhalation to move the abdominal muscles outward, has been shown to be the best form of breathing to relieve stress. Chest breathing tends to be shallower and more rapid and is commonly practiced when a person is under stress.

In order to learn abdominal breathing, it is best to lie on your back and place a large book, such as a dictionary, phone book, or a large family Bible, on the abdomen. While breathing, move the abdomen outward, thus causing the book to rise higher in the air. Concentrate on moving the abdomen outward and not expanding the rib cage or upper chest area.

As this is practiced, you will be able to perform abdominal

breathing while sitting, standing, or walking. When you feel stressed, perform five or ten slow, deep abdominal breaths to relax your body.

Progressive Muscle Relaxation Exercises

Practice this when you are reclining in a comfortable chair, on a bed, or on the couch. Close your eyes to relax. Beginning with your feet, tense your toes by curling them under; hold this position for five seconds and then relax. As you relax, simply allow the tension to leave your body.

Next, flex your ankle joints. With your legs flat on the bed, couch, or floor, pull your toes and feet back while flexing your calf muscles. Again, hold this position for five seconds and then relax.

Next, point your toes like a ballerina, and again flex your calves for five seconds. Move to your legs and flex your thighs tight. Hold this for five seconds and relax.

Gradually working your way up your body, flex the muscles in your abdomen, arms, chest, shoulders, hands, neck, forehead, eyes, and jaw. Once again, do each of these for five seconds and then relax. The tension will actually melt away.

A **Bible Cure** Health Tip
Heat Therapy

Heat therapy is ideal for most people with fibromyalgia. Depending on how severe your pain is, you can try either surface heat (hot packs, heating pads) that heats the skin only, or deep heat (whirlpool baths, paraffin waxing) that heats all the way down to the core of your muscles. If exercising leaves you stiff or sore, try some heat therapy before and afterward.

STRETCHING

Stretching is the perfect place to begin your exercise routine because it will help improve the symptoms of CFS and fibromyalgia while it builds up your endurance at the same time. Stretching elongates the muscles, which helps to relieve the stiffness. This along with deep breathing helps to deliver nutrients and oxygen to the tissues and remove metabolic waste products that build up from poor blood flow due to chronic muscle tension. It also increases your flexibility, which helps give you a broader range of motions for all sorts of everyday tasks and activities. Last but not least, it helps you fall asleep faster and be less likely to wake up during the night.

Stretching is good for everyone, but if you are suffering from the symptoms of chronic fatigue or fibromyalgia, there are a few things you should keep in mind:

- Get your muscles ready to stretch by taking a warm bath or shower or using a heating pad or hot packs right before your stretching session. If you are particularly stiff or sore, do your stretches while you are in a warm bath or whirlpool. (Don't try to do stretches while standing in the shower; it's too easy to slip and fall.)

- Hold a stretch until you feel a good deal of resistance, but never to the point of pain. Don't bounce while stretching, or you may tear a muscle. If a certain muscle is sore, do fewer repetitions of that stretch or hold it for a shorter length of time.

- Ask a friend to help you if you are having trouble holding your stretches. You will get the same benefit whether you do your stretches alone or

with help. If you don't enjoy exercising alone, try
a beginner stretching class, such as beginner's yoga
or Pilates.

- Start slow, doing only one rep of each stretch and
holding it for a short amount of time. Build very,
very gradually. If you push too hard, you can
aggravate your condition and end up feeling even
worse.

- Don't forget to focus on your breathing while you
stretch, making sure to breathe deeply, and never
hold your breath. Remember, you are delivering
oxygen to muscles that are literally starving for it
due to restricted blood flow from chronic muscle
tension and spasms.

I provide descriptions and photos of an entire stretching routine
you can try at home in chapter 10 of my book *Get Fit and Live!*

START A REGULAR WALKING ROUTINE

The next exercise to build into your routine after you've incorporated
some good stretches is walking. The key is to start slowly and
gradually build your walking routine.

Walking can be a very enjoyable exercise because you can
incorporate it with many other interests. If you love the outdoors,
take a slow walk through your favorite park. If shopping is your
thing, then take a slow walk through the mall and window shop.

Start with a five-minute walk every other day and gradually
increase your speed and time as tolerated. Initially I recommend
that you exercise every other day instead of daily until your body
adjusts to the schedule. If your fatigue or fibromyalgia becomes

worse, then simply decrease your intensity (slow down) and decrease your exercise time; over time you will be able to exercise five days a week, and you will get healthier and stronger.

Many prefer to walk for five minutes twice a day rather than ten minutes once a day. This is perfectly acceptable. Eventually, work your way up to a ten- to fifteen-minute walk twice a day (or a twenty- to thirty-minute walk once a day), if you are able, but be very careful not to push yourself too fast.

A **BIBLE CURE** *Health Tip*
Stop to Address Adrenal Fatigue

If you begin a simple walking routine but find that it causes complete exhaustion, you may have very low adrenal function due to long-term chronic stress. If this is the case, you should refrain from walking or any other form of aerobic exercise until your adrenal function has been adequately restored. Rest and take the supplements that will be discussed in chapter 6 to restore adrenal function. By following the other Bible Cure steps to restore adrenal function, you will eventually be able to perform moderate exercise without exhaustion.

Just as you should never push yourself if stretching or exercise causes pain, you also should never push yourself if you feel exhausted after exercise. You could further deplete your adrenal glands and cause even severer fatigue. Use balance and wisdom.

ADD AEROBIC EXERCISE WHEN
YOU'RE READY FOR MORE

Your fatigue may not be at such a severe level. If so, you may be able to work through the earlier building stages more quickly and eventually get into more vigorous exercise. (Before adding aerobic exercise of any kind to your routine, please check with your doctor.) I typically recommend that you work your way up to exercising for twenty to thirty minutes every other day—and eventually increasing this to every day, five days a week—at 65 percent of your maximum heart rate (see the Bible Cure Health Tip below) when battling mild fibromyalgia and chronic fatigue.

A **BIBLE CURE** *Health Tip*
Your Predicted Heart Rate

Calculate your target heart rate zone using this formula:

220 minus [your age] = _____

x .65 = _____

(This is your recommended heart rate. However, as your body starts to heal, you will be able to gradually increase your intensity.)

This example may help: To calculate the target heart zone for a forty-year-old woman with CFS or fibromyalgia, subtract the age (40) from 220 (220 – 40 = 180). Multiply 180 by .65, which equals 117. A 40-year-old woman's target heart rate is 117 beats per minute.

When your body starts to heal, you will be able to increase your target heart rate. Eventually you may be able to go up to 80 percent of your maximum heart rate. In the example of the forty-year-old woman above, 80 percent would equal 144 beats per minute.

Of course, you'll want to increase your activity at a slow pace. I also recommend you always warm up and cool down with stretches. Keep in mind that you might feel some discomfort as you increase your activity level or try new activities; everyone does. This should subside as your body adjusts to the new activities. If you've mastered stretching and walking and feel you're ready for additional aerobic activities, check with your doctor about the following recommendations:

- Water—either swimming or a water aerobics class; you don't need to know how to swim to take water aerobics; you can wear a floatation device if needed.

- Cycling—either outdoors or on a stationary bike; work your way up from five to thirty minutes, two or three times a week. If you have neck or back pain, look for a recumbent (upright) stationary cycle.

WHEN YOU'RE READY: TRY REBOUNDING EXERCISES

Eventually when your fatigue and fibromyalgia pain and other symptoms are improved, one of the best exercises for both CFS and fibromyalgia is rebounding (jumping on a mini-trampoline) because both of these disorders are associated with poor lymphatic flow.

The lymphatic system is a major microbe fighter and cellular garbage collector in the body. It removes toxins and cellular waste as well as killing viruses and bacteria. Your body contains three times more lymph than blood, but the lymphatic system has a challenge: it is circulated by muscle contractions and not your heartbeat. When you don't move, your lymphatic system becomes sluggish. Aerobic exercise can triple the rate of your lymphatic flow. However, the best exercise to improve lymphatic flow is rebounding.

Albert E. Carter, author of *Rebound Exercise: The Ultimate Exercise for the New Millennium*, has experienced firsthand the various health benefits of rebounding throughout his life. He can perform one hundred push-ups and has never lifted weights in his life. He taught both of his children to rebound from a very early age. His son, Darren, was able to do 429 sit-ups the first time he was challenged (in the first grade), and his daughter, Wendie, was able to do 476 sit-ups without stopping and beat all the boys in her sixth grade class in arm wrestling even though she had never arm wrestled before![1] It's interesting that the only exercise they did was to jump on a trampoline.

I highly recommend this form of exercise not only for CFS and fibromyalgia sufferers, but also for its benefits in fighting cancer due to the way it improves lymphatic flow. I provide a complete seven-minute rebounding routine, along with important rebounding safety tips, in my book *Get Fit and Live!*

A Word of Caution

For CFS and fibromyalgia sufferers, I do NOT recommend initially starting any strengthening exercises (also called anaerobic or resistance exercises). The strengthening exercises come much later when your fatigue and painful trigger points are resolved or much improved.

Toning and strengthening exercises will many times worsen both chronic fatigue and fibromyalgia. The reason is that toning and strengthening will typically make the muscle spasms experienced by fibromyalgia sufferers worse. Also, people with chronic fatigue usually have adrenal fatigue, which is like an overdrawn bank account. (Refer to chapter 6 for supplements that can address adrenal fatigue.) I also discuss adrenal fatigue at greater length in my books *Stress Less* and *The New Bible Cure for Stress*. Toning and resistance exercises—and even too much aerobic exercise—will further deplete energy levels or adrenal reserves, possibly making the symptoms of CFS and fibromyalgia worse.

In summary, the kind of exercise and frequency that will be right for you will depend on the severity of your symptoms of chronic fatigue syndrome or fibromyalgia. And remember, it's OK to start slow because as you perform the stretches and aerobics described in this chapter, you will improve lymphatic flow and help to relax your muscles, which should improve your condition.

ADDITIONAL TIPS

Here are some additional tips to help you stick with it.

- First, don't look at exercise as something you can do in your spare time. Make this time an important part of your day.

- Second, if you don't enjoy exercising alone, get an exercise buddy or join a class. In addition, don't think about it as work.

- Third, remember to give yourself extra time to rest and recover after any new activity. Be patient while your body begins to build strength and endurance over time.

- And lastly, see exercise as a special time to be alone with God, surrounded by the wonders of His creation. As you exercise, thank God for all of His love for you and for His blessings in your life.

> The LORD gives his people strength. The LORD blesses
> them with peace.
>
> —PSALM 29:11

CONCLUSION

With God's help in taking these simple, practical steps, you can reduce stress and its accompanying fatigue and pain while increasing strength and vitality. If you find yourself under constant stress in the world's fast-paced system, then take comfort in this Bible Cure promise: "For this good news—that God has prepared this rest—has been announced to us just as it was to them" (Heb. 4:2). Rest isn't just for individuals who lived during Bible times. God's rest is for you right now.

A **BIBLE CURE** Prayer for You

Heavenly Father, help me reduce the stress in my life that robs my vitality and saps my strength. Show me how to work with more wisdom instead of working in ways that foolishly waste my strength. Fill me with Your peace and rest so that I may be renewed by Your presence and power. Thank You for giving me the peace that passes all understanding. Amen.

A BIBLE CURE *Prescription*

Check the ways you will begin reducing your stress and symptoms of CFS and fibromyalgia:

❏ Get proper rest and relaxation.

❏ Practice abdominal breathing.

❏ Use muscle relaxation exercises.

❏ Begin a stretching routine.

❏ Begin a slow walking routine and gradually increase it.

❏ Add more aerobic exercise as tolerated.

Chapter 5

RENEW WITH REST

G OD PLANS TO renew you, strengthen you, and refresh you with rest. If you feel completely drained, tired, and spent, you may have some doubts about that. Stop looking at the enormity of your fatigue and begin seeing the greatness of God.

Consider God's promise to you:

> Have you never heard? Have you never understood? The LORD is the everlasting God, the Creator of all the earth. He never grows weak or weary. No one can measure the depths of his understanding. He gives power to the weak and strength to the powerless. Even youths will become weak and tired, and young men will fall in exhaustion. But those who trust in the LORD will find new strength. They will soar high on wings like eagles. They will run and not grow weary. They will walk and not faint.
>
> —ISAIAH 40:28–31

This promise is for you. You will run and not grow weary when you put your trust in God. What a wonderful promise, and what a wonderful God! He is so great that He created the universe, but He is greater still because He sees you, right there in your circumstances, and He cares for you with a love that knows no limits. He will get you through this, and you will feel good once more. Isn't that great news?

ARE YOU GETTING YOUR REST?

When my son was in high school, he played golf. However, he would often forget to charge his golf cart, and it would suddenly run out of juice. He would have to push it to the nearest place where he could charge it. Our bodies are very similar. If we do not adequately recharge our bodies with enough deep, restful sleep, our minds and our bodies will become extremely fatigued and will burn out before the end of the day.

During sleep, our bodies are repairing tissues that have been damaged or excessively stressed during the waking hours of the day. When you do not rest properly, your body becomes fatigued very quickly.

While many people do not know how much sleep they actually need, most need, on average, about seven to eight hours every night. Some people, however, may manage on just five or six hours, while others may need as many as ten hours of sleep a night.

Women usually need to sleep longer than men. Elderly patients usually sleep less as they age. However, they still require about seven to eight hours of sleep a night. Often the reduction in sleep experienced by the elderly is because the sleep hormone, melatonin, decreases with age.

Our bodies need sleep to resist disease, maintain strength and endurance, increase vitality, improve our moods, and even slow down aging. Deep, restful sleep and adequate dreaming will fully restore our bodies and our brains, thus improving our intellectual abilities, our moods, our emotional strength, and even our attitudes.

God is able to give you rest and restore your strength when

you are weary. He will also help you discover the cause of your sleeplessness. Even if you are experiencing mild or severe depression, which can cause countless sleepless nights, the Bible cure will help. A number of natural ways for you to rest and overcome fatigue are available to you. Let me explore those ways with you.

A BIBLE CURE *Health Tip*
If You Have Trouble Sleeping

Aerobic exercise, such as walking, swimming, or cycling during the day (but not within a few hours of bedtime), may improve your quality of sleep. Regular aerobic exercise helps your body to make smooth transitions between sleep cycles and stages of sleep. See chapter 4 for information on exercise.

AVOID SLEEPING PILLS

When individuals have trouble falling asleep or staying asleep, often they go to their doctor to get some sleeping pills. But did you know that many sleeping pills, especially benzodiazepines, actually tend to disrupt normal sleep? Sleeping pills interrupt the natural REM sleep cycle we spoke of earlier, as well as the deeper stages of non-REM sleep.

Therefore, sleeping pills can only help you receive superficial sleep. You may get more hours of sleep, but you typically won't enter the deeper stages of sleep. You probably will wake up groggy and usually will feel fatigued throughout the day.

Over-the-counter sleep medications and medications containing antihistamines, such as Benadryl, also commonly cause fatigue throughout the day.

Insomnia is simply difficulty falling asleep or difficulty staying asleep. Doctors think of it in terms of sleep-onset insomnia (difficulty falling asleep) and sleep-maintenance insomnia (difficulty staying there). The most common causes of sleep-onset insomnia are stress, anxiety, caffeine, alcohol, pain or discomfort, or change in environment. Common causes of sleep-maintenance insomnia include depression, low blood sugar, nocturnal leg cramps, pain, alcohol, and changes in environment.

ELIMINATE STIMULANTS

An important step in getting a good night's sleep is eliminating stimulants such as caffeine, decongestants, and diet pills. These drugs will alter the normal architecture of sleep, preventing you from reaching the deep stages of sleep. They will also alter rapid eye movements, which will decrease your dreaming and cause fragmented sleep and increased fatigue.

Since a good night's sleep is probably the single most important factor in preventing fatigue, you should avoid or decrease substances that cause insomnia. Caffeine is a powerful stimulant that arouses the body and actually activates the nerves and muscles. Caffeine is found in coffee, tea, soft drinks, chocolate, hot chocolate, certain medications, and even coffee-flavored ice cream.

If you choose to drink caffeinated beverages, I recommend limiting them to breakfast or lunch. Avoid consuming caffeinated foods and beverages at dinner or before bedtime. If you have any liver impairment, which may occur when taking statin drugs that lower cholesterol, you are likely especially sensitive to the effects of caffeine and should only consume it at breakfast, if at all.

A **BIBLE CURE** Health Fact
Caffeine

- The average amount of caffeine in a cup of coffee ranges from approximately 100–150 mg.
- The average amount of caffeine in a 12-ounce glass of tea is 70 mg.
- 7-Up, Sprite, and most clear soft drinks have no caffeine.
- Mountain Dew (12 ounces) has approximately 54 mg of caffeine.
- Coke Classic (12 ounces) has approximately 35 mg of caffeine.
- Pepsi (12 ounces) has approximately 38 mg of caffeine.
- Jolt (12 ounces) has approximately 72 mg of caffeine.[1]

Caffeine will actually block the effects of serotonin and melatonin, which are two very important chemicals in the brain that cause you to fall asleep and remain asleep. If you are having difficulty sleeping, the first thing you should do is limit your caffeine consumption to a small amount at breakfast. If you still have trouble sleeping, I recommend you eliminate all caffeine from your diet for a while to see if your sleep improves.

AVOID ALCOHOL

Alcohol is another chemical that can cause sleep disturbances. Many people think that a glass of wine at night will help relax them and help them fall asleep. Alcohol actually causes our bodies to release adrenaline, which gets us ready for "fight or flight," therefore stimulating our bodies.

Alcohol may decrease tryptophan levels in the brain, which leads to lower serotonin levels and, as a result, may cause sleep disturbances. Alcohol will also delay and actually decrease the REM stage of sleep, causing a person to sleep lightly and feel tired and groggy during the day.

EARLY TO BED

Do you go to bed after the evening news near midnight, after first falling asleep in front of the television set? Break late-night habits. Go to bed as early in the evening as possible, and strive to get at least eight hours of sleep each night. Establish a regular bedtime, preferable around 9:30 to 10:00 p.m. A regular bedtime even on the weekends and holidays is the most important sleep habit to develop if you have chronic fatigue and fibromyalgia. If an afternoon nap interferes with your sleep at night, then you should limit your nap to only thirty minute or less, or stop taking a nap altogether.

A BIBLE CURE *Health Tip*
Top Sleep Hygiene Recommendations

"Sleep hygiene" is simply establishing healthy sleep habits. I recommend the following twenty-five sleep hygiene habits that will enable most people to fall asleep and stay asleep.

1. Establish a regular bedtime and waking up time—and stick to this routine even on weekends and vacations.
2. Use your bed only for sleep and intimacy with your spouse (not for reading, watching TV, snacking, working, etc.).

3. Avoid naps after 3:00 p.m. and limit them to twenty or thirty minutes.

4. Exercise before dinner.

5. Avoid caffeine in the afternoon and evening.

6. Avoid drinking excessive fluids in the late evening and before bedtime.

7. Eat normal portions of a well-balanced meal for dinner, at least three hours before bedtime, and a light, well-balanced bedtime snack.

8. Take a warm bath one to two hours before bed, adding a few drops of lavender oil for help with relaxation.

9. Keep the bedroom cool and well ventilated.

10. Purchase a comfortable mattress, pillow, and linens.

11. Thirty minutes before going to bed, start to wind down by listening to soothing music, reading, having a massage, or being intimate with your spouse.

12. Put dimmer switches on your lights and dim them a few hours prior to bedtime.

13. If you are not asleep within twenty minutes of lying down, simply get up, go into another room, and read or relax in dim lights until you feel sleepy. Then return to bed.

14. If your spouse frequently awakens you with snoring or unusual movements, move to another bed such as in a guest bedroom.

15. Exchange foot, neck, shoulder, and back massages with your spouse.

16. Relax your mind and body before bedtime with gentle stretching or relaxation exercises.

17. Burn aromatherapy candles or oils before bedtime to aid with relaxation.

18. Clean clutter out of the bedroom. Remove all computers, fax machines, paperwork, and anything that reminds you of work.

19. Make sure your bedroom is completely dark. Remove nightlights, and cover alarm clocks and phone lights with a towel. Cover other visible lights on alarm systems, stereos, TVs, DVD players, etc. with black electrical tape or sticky notes. Purchase blackout curtains or blinds.

20. If your spouse or children must turn on lights in the bedroom, bathroom, closet, or hallway while you are trying to sleep, wear a sleep mask to block these lights.

21. Block out noise with earplugs, double-pane windows, heavy drapes, or a fan. You can also purchase sound generators that will play white noise or relaxing sounds to help you fall asleep.

22. Keep pets out of your bedroom. In addition to snoring, pouncing, growling, howling, or barking, they can trigger allergies in some people.

23. Avoid watching heart-pounding movies, ball games, or late-night news. Instead, watch something funny or lighthearted before bed.

24. Avoid watching television in the bedroom or falling asleep with the television on.

25. Memorize and meditate on Scripture if you awaken during the night, and do not let your mind worry or wander.

RESTLESS LEG SYNDROME

Restless leg syndrome is another cause of chronic fatigue. It is closely related to nocturnal myoclonus. Restless leg syndrome is simply that: restlessness of the legs. During sleep, an individual with restless leg syndrome has a strong urge to move his legs. Nocturnal myoclonus is characterized by jerking movements or muscle contractions of leg muscles while asleep. The restless legs and the contractions, cramping, and jerking of the leg muscles may happen frequently throughout the night, causing insomnia and sleep disturbances that eventually result in extreme fatigue and exhaustion.

An iron deficiency can contribute to restless leg syndrome. Rule this out by getting your doctor to test your serum ferritin level, which measures how much iron your body has stored.

If the above measures fail to relieve the symptoms of restless leg syndrome, I recommend that you try supplementing with 5-HTP, magnesium, melatonin, L-tryptophan, L-theanine, or chamomile tea before bed. (See Appendix B.) I also recommend you try the twenty-five sleep hygiene habits I've listed in this chapter.

SLEEP APNEA

Sleep apnea affects over 18 million Americans, and approximately 10 million Americans are not even diagnosed. Over 50 percent of all the patients with sleep apnea are over forty years of age. Sleep apnea is more common in men than women, with 4–9 percent of middle-aged men with apnea and only 2–4 percent of middle-aged women with apnea.[2]

Sleep apnea is associated with severe fatigue and daytime sleepiness, memory loss, irritability, accidents, and premature death. People with sleep apnea usually have problems with concentration, reaction time, and learning. Their brains have been deprived of oxygen, and they are usually simply exhausted from the lack of quality sleep.

Continued oxygen deprivation puts a strain on the heart and lungs and eventually may raise the blood pressure as the vital organs are literally being starved of oxygen. This is why people with sleep apnea have an increased risk of hypertension, heart problems (including heart attacks and cardiac arrest), type 2 diabetes, and even depression.

In order to diagnose sleep apnea, you need to undergo a sleep study at a sleep lab. Sleep apnea is usually treated with CPAP (continuous positive airway pressure) or BiPAP (bilevel positive airway pressure). AVAPS (average volume assured pressure support) is a new technology in treating sleep apnea introduced into the United States in 2007. It ensures an adequate depth of breathing and is a special feature to some BiPAP machines. Weight loss and especially decreasing your neck size are often useful in relieving or decreasing the severity of sleep apnea. Somnoplasty may also benefit those with mild apnea. More information on sleep apnea and other sleep disorders can be found in my book *The New Bible Cure for Sleep Disorders*.

> But LORD, be merciful to us, for we have waited for you. Be our strong arm each day and our salvation in times of trouble.
>
> —ISAIAH 33:2

LOW BLOOD SUGAR

Most people with chronic fatigue and fibromyalgia are prone to develop hypoglycemia (low blood sugar) during the night since low blood sugar is very common in patients with adrenal fatigue; most all patients with chronic fatigue and fibromyalgia have adrenal fatigue. As a result, they have restless sleep. When the blood sugar level drops, the body releases certain hormones to raise the blood sugar as rapidly as possible. These hormones include adrenaline, cortisol, and glycogen. As a result, the brain tells the body it's time to eat and may jolt the body awake. By simply eating a well-balanced protein and carb bedtime snack (for example: plain or vanilla Greek yogurt with some nuts; a slice of turkey and high-fiber crackers; or a small serving of beans and brown rice), you will usually prevent low blood sugar during the night. These carbohydrates will help to raise the level of serotonin, which will keep you sleeping soundly.

If you have candida, you should avoid gluten and yogurt. Eat a small serving of beans and brown rice, turkey and brown rice, or almond or rice crackers with some hummus or almond butter instead.

CONCLUSION

The Bible Cure pathway to decreasing fatigue and increasing your strength and energy daily is to get enough sleep. It's time for you to rest in the Lord and let go of habits and overcome physical problems that interrupt your sleep.

God promises to give you rest and increase your strength. Your Bible Cure promise is found in the well-known Twenty-Third Psalm. I have adapted that psalm as a Bible Cure prayer for you to pray daily as you seek His rest and strength.

A **BIBLE CURE** Prayer for You

Lord, You are my shepherd; I have everything I need. Thank You for letting me rest in green meadows and leading me beside peaceful streams. I praise You for renewing my strength. Lord, guide me along right paths, that I might bring honor to Your name. Even when I walk through the dark valley of death, I will not be afraid, for You are close beside me. Your rod and Your staff protect and comfort me. You prepare a feast for me in the presence of my enemies. You welcome me as a guest, anointing my head with oil. My cup overflows with blessings. Surely Your goodness and unfailing love will pursue me all the days of my life, and I will live in the house of the Lord forever. Amen.

—*Adapted from Psalm 23*

A **BIBLE CURE** Prescription

In order to rest properly, you must limit or eliminate certain things in your life. Check those things below that you will limit or eliminate:

❏ Caffeine
❏ Sleeping pills
❏ Alcohol

Check the positive steps you will take:

❏ Get seven to eight hours of sleep regularly.
❏ Go to bed at a regular time.

Thank God for His rest, care, and peace in your life.

Chapter 6

RESTORE WITH VITAMINS
AND SUPPLEMENTS

Your body is a masterful balance of artistry and chemistry, a perfect design of creative genius. God alone could create you—and He intricately and wonderfully made you! The Bible states, "You made all the delicate, inner parts of my body and knit me together in my mother's womb. Thank you for making me so wonderfully complex! Your workmanship is marvelous—how well I know it. You watched me as I was being formed in utter seclusion, as I was woven together in the dark of the womb" (Ps. 139:13–15).

The divine Creator has also supplied countless sources of energy to restore, strengthen, and nourish this wonderful machine. Vitamins and minerals are uniquely programmed by God to support the various systems of your body.

God desires for you to take care of your body, the temple of God's Spirit, so that you can live a fully abundant life serving Him. Although found in some measure in the foods we eat, supplemental vitamins and minerals will both strengthen your body and give you the vitality you need to overcome fatigue.

Don't be discouraged. Don't quit, and don't give up. You will win out over fatigue! Trust His promise: "But those who trust in the LORD will find new strength. They will soar high on wings like eagles. They will run and not grow weary. They will walk and not faint" (Isa. 40:31).

> This is what the Sovereign LORD, the Holy One of Israel, says: "Only in returning to me and resting in me will you be saved. In quietness and confidence is your strength."
>
> —ISAIAH 30:15

SUPPLEMENTS FOR ADRENAL FATIGUE*

Since most patients with fibromyalgia and chronic fatigue have significant adrenal fatigue, I always place them on supplements that support the adrenal glands. There are many types of supplements to help support and restore the adrenal glands, but I will list here my favorite supplements for adrenal fatigue, especially for those suffering from fibromyalgia and chronic fatigue syndrome.

1. *A multivitamin.* Take a comprehensive multivitamin that contains adequate amounts of magnesium, niacin, and B_6, which are important cofactors in converting 5-HTP to serotonin.

2. *B-complex vitamins.* For many years the B vitamins have been known as the "stress relief" vitamins. The B vitamins provide the greatest benefit when they are supplemented together, such as a balanced B "complex." Some B vitamins actually require other B

---

* If you are pregnant, nursing, taking any prescription drugs, or are allergic to any of the ingredients, please consult with your health care practitioner prior to use.

vitamins for activation. The B vitamins are especially important for elderly individuals since B vitamins are not absorbed as well as a person ages. The B vitamins are associated primarily with the brain and nervous system function and are used in the production of ATP. Deficiency in any or all of them is commonly associated with fatigue and sleep disturbances, eventually resulting in atrophy of the adrenal glands. Vitamin B_5 (pantothenic acid) is especially important because it plays a significant part in the production of adrenal hormones; it is sometimes called the antistress vitamin. I recommend taking a B-complex vitamin two to three times a day. (See Appendix B.)

3. *Minerals.* The human body also needs twenty-two essential minerals on a daily basis. Many people are deficient in several of these minerals. There are seven major minerals: calcium, phosphorus, sodium, chloride, magnesium, potassium, and sulfur. Of these major minerals, many people are deficient in calcium and magnesium. We also need fifteen trace minerals: boron, chromium, cobalt, copper, fluoride, iodine, iron, manganese, molybdenum, nickel, selenium, silicon, tin, vanadium, and zinc. Because our soil has become depleted or is lacking in minerals, the food we grow and eat provides less and less of these essential nutrients. Therefore, the vast majority of Americans need to take minerals in supplement form.

   Stress and high cortisol levels also cause depletion of certain nutrients in the body. People who are under excessive stress nearly always need to have an increase in the B vitamins, vitamin C, magnesium, zinc, copper, chromium, selenium, and vitamin E.

Low magnesium levels are very common in individuals with adrenal fatigue. Approximately three-fourths of the US population does not consume adequate amounts of magnesium in their diets. Increased stress as well as adrenal fatigue cause our bodies to have an increased need for magnesium. Magnesium is involved in the activation of more than three hundred enzymes in the body. It is vital to health. When cortisol and adrenaline levels are elevated, there is also an increase of urinary excretion of magnesium. This indicates that in times of stress, our bodies have an increased need for magnesium. The dietary recommendation for magnesium is 300 mg. I commonly recommend 200 mg of magnesium two times a day. (See Appendix B.)

4. *DHEA* is involved in many processes in the human body. It promotes the growth and repair of protein tissue, especially muscle, and it acts to regulate cortisol, negating many of the harmful effects of ongoing excessive cortisol. When demands for cortisol are increased for a prolonged time, DHEA levels decline and the DHEA no longer is able to balance the negative effects of excess cortisol. A depressed level of DHEA may serve as an early warning sign of adrenal exhaustion.

After age twenty-five, DHEA levels begin to decline. By the time a person is sixty years old, he has only about a quarter of the DHEA he had when he was twenty. By the time he is eighty, he has only about 20 percent of what he had when he was sixty.

I have found that DHEA liposomal cream is a superior delivery system for DHEA and delivers adequate amounts of DHEA throughout the day and night. I recommend three pumps for women and five pumps for men with fibromyalgia and/or chronic fatigue, once or twice a day. Apply it to the full length of one arm and rub it in. (See Appendix B.)

5. *Pregnenolone.* If DHEA is considered the "mother" hormone, then pregnenolone is the "grandmother" hormone. It is a natural hormone discovered in the 1940s and is made largely from cholesterol, which is used, in turn, to make DHEA. When the body is under stress, pregnenolone is used to produce more cortisol.

Pregnenolone is one of the most effective and powerful memory boosters and may help to prevent memory loss and dementia. It is known as the "hormone balancer" since it has the ability to increase levels of steroid hormones that are deficient in the body and can decrease excessive levels of circulating hormones. Supplementation can be beneficial for many people who experiencing the symptoms of chronic fatigue and fibromyalgia. I again recommend the pregnenolone liposomal cream in a dose of three pumps for women and five pumps for men with fibromyalgia and/or chronic fatigue, once or twice a day, applied to the full length of the arm and rubbed in. (See Appendix B.)

6. *Adrenal glandular supplements* contain protomorphogens or extracts of tissues from the adrenal glands of pigs or cattle. These can be taken orally to support human adrenal function. Each

organ of the body has a unique mix of vitamins, minerals, and hormones. Glandular substances in pigs and cattle have an "adrenal mix" close to that of the human adrenal glands. Some doctors of natural medicine have used adrenal glandular supplements with their patients for decades and report very positive results. (See Appendix B.)

7. *Progesterone (for women).* As women age, the ovaries gradually produce less and less progesterone, and eventually the production ceases around menopause. In even younger women suffering from severe adrenal fatigue, cortisol levels are typically low, as are progesterone levels. This is because the body robs progesterone from the ovaries to produce cortisol, which becomes depleted under long-term stress. Some women benefit from bioidentical progesterone supplementation using transdermal creams or an oral dose of progesterone at bedtime if the patient has insomnia. If women test low for female hormones, I recommend a bioidentical progesterone cream. This is a prescription and must be prescribed by a physician. (See Appendix B.)

8. *Adaptogens.* An adaptogen is a substance that will help the body adapt to stress by balancing cortisol levels. They help the body's mental and physical performance while providing resistance to stressful insults at the cellular level. Adaptogens include rhodiola, Korean ginseng, Siberian ginseng, ashwagandha, and epimedium. More information can be found in my book *Stress Less*. (See Appendix B for recommended products.)

SUPPLEMENTS FOR ENERGY

Over-the-counter energy supplements such as caffeine and most energy drinks usually stress the adrenal glands, but I have found a few key supplements that increase one's energy without stressing and draining adrenal function.

1. *Glutathione-boosting supplements.* Glutathione is known as the master antioxidant in the body and functions as a detoxifier of the body, neutralizing toxins and heavy metals as well as quenching free radicals. Its helps to maintain your body's energy-producing mitochondria and enables the mitochondria to produce optimal amounts of ATP by quenching free radicals. ATP is the energy currency in the body.

   Glutathione is produced in your body and recycled by your body all the time—except chronic diseases, including CFS and fibromyalgia, usually deplete the glutathione in our bodies. Also, glutathione levels typically decrease by 1 percent per year after age twenty-one. But I find that CFS and fibromyalgia patients usually have very low levels of glutathione and as a consequence very low energy. If oxidative stress or toxins overwhelm your body, your glutathione levels drop and your body's protection against free radicals, infections, and illnesses becomes greatly compromised. It becomes harder for your body to get rid of the toxins as well. This creates a vicious cycle of chronic illness.

   Studies have found that people with chronic fatigue syndrome are usually depleted in glutathione, and boosting their intracellular glutathione levels may help their symptoms improve.[1]

I recommend glutathione-boosting supplements to every patient with chronic fatigue or fibromyalgia. (See Appendix B.)

2. *D-ribose.* D-ribose is a simple 5-carbon sugar that helps build new ATP. Supplementing with D-ribose in one study increased the total amount of ATP produced by up to fourfold.[2] I recommend usually one scoop two times a day in water or green tea. (See Appendix B.)

3. *Acetyl L-carnitine and alpha lipoic acid.* Acetyl L-carnitine boosts the conversion of fats into energy in the mitochondria. Alpha lipoic acid is also involved in mitochondrial ATP production and can recycle other antioxidants. Together they work synergistically. I recommend 1,000–2,000 mg daily for acetyl L-carnitine and 20–50 mg daily of alpha lipoic acid. (See Appendix B.)

4. *NADH* increases energy significantly and may help to enhance the immune system, fighting disease and repairing damage caused by the disease. I recommend 5–10 mg, two times a day. (See Appendix B.)

5. *Coenzyme Q_{10}* helps increase ATP (energy) and is especially effective when combined with PQQ (below). Ubiquinol is the biologically superior form of CoQ_{10}. I recommend 50 mg, two times a day. (See Appendix B.)

6. *Pyrroloquinoline quinone (PQQ)* is an antioxidant compound that is emerging as the micronutrient that may reverse cellular aging. It plays an essential role in

defending cells against mitochondrial decay. PQQ's chemical structure enables it to withstand exposure to oxidation up to five thousand times greater than vitamin C. It not only protects mitochondria from damage, but it also stimulates growth of new mitochondria. I recommend 20 mg per day. (See Appendix B.)

7. *Myers IV.* The Myers IV helps to restore adrenal function. Nutrients in a Myers IV include magnesium chloride, calcium gluconate, methylcobalamin, pyridoxine hydrochloride, pantothenic acid, vitamin B_6, vitamin B_5, B-complex, and buffered vitamin C. I usually give this IV to my patients with chronic fatigue and fibromyalgia. (See Appendix B.)

SUPPLEMENTS TO HELP YOU SLEEP

Listed below are supplements that will help relieve insomnia and produce a good quality sleep.

1. *L-tryptophan and its metabolite 5-HTP* (5-hydroxytryptophan) are forms of tryptophan, which is an amino acid that is a step closer to forming the neurotransmitter serotonin. Serotonin is extremely important in both improving the quality of your sleep and helping you to fall asleep.

    5-HTP actually improves the quality of sleep by increasing the time spent in REM sleep and also by increasing the time spent in stages three and four of phase one, which are the deeper stages of sleep. The amount of time spent in superficial sleep, stages one and two, is actually decreased. However, these are the least important stages of sleep. The total time of sleep is not prolonged. In other words, you will spend more time in deeper sleep and have more time in REM sleep, causing more dreaming and thus awaken more refreshed.

Like the example of recharging a golf cart, if you were able to improve both your sleep quality and the time spent in REM sleep, you would be able to fully charge your physical and mental batteries. This would provide more energy, mental clarity, and possibly even more creativity during the day.

Normally, I recommend approximately 100 to 300 mg of 5-HTP thirty minutes to an hour prior to going to bed. Higher doses of 5-HTP can sometimes produce nightmares; therefore, start low and gradually increase the dosage until sleep quality has improved. The dosage for L-tryptophan is one to three tablets, 500 mg, at bedtime. However, I prefer 5-HTP.

2. *L-theanine and GABA.* Elevated stress hormones, especially cortisol, eventually disrupt brain chemistry and cause imbalances in neurotransmitters, including serotonin, dopamine, norepinephrine, and GABA, as well as other brain chemicals.

However, the amino acid L-theanine crosses the blood-brain barrier and is able to suppress stress hormones, including cortisol. L-theanine helps the body to produce other calming neurotransmitters, including GABA, serotonin, and dopamine.

I find that L-theanine typically works better with GABA, so I frequently prescribe these two supplements be taken together with vitamin B_6 to help calm the mind as well as lower the stress hormones and help you fall asleep. I usually recommend 200–400 mg of L-theanine with 500–1,000 mg of GABA at bedtime taken with vitamin B_6. This combination may also be taken with melatonin and 5-HTP or L-tryptophan. For more information on GABA, please see *The New Bible Cure for Depression and Anxiety.*

3. *Melatonin* is a hormone secreted by the pineal gland. It is important in both helping you fall asleep and maintaining your sleep. I normally start with a dose of 1 to 3 mg of melatonin at bedtime. I may gradually increase that dose to 20 mg at bedtime and 10 mg if they awaken during the night. (See Appendix B.)

4. *Chamomile and other teas.* For centuries people have used chamomile tea to treat insomnia. Chamomile tea is a mild muscle relaxant and has mild sedative properties; it may also help relieve stress, anxiety, and depression. It usually helps promote a deep sleep as well as feelings of relaxation and calmness. The active ingredients are oils found in the flowers of chamomile. Sleepytime Tea is a brand of tea that blends chamomile, spearmint, and lemongrass. There is also Sleepytime Extra, which adds valerian. A word of caution: if you are allergic to ragweed, you should avoid chamomile and Sleepytime Tea. (For more teas, see Appendix B.)

> I am praying to you because I know you will answer, O God. Bend down and listen as I pray. Show me your unfailing love in wonderful ways. By your mighty power you rescue those who seek refuge from their enemies. Guard me as you would guard your own eyes. Hide me in the shadow of your wings.
>
> —Psalm 17:6–8

TREATING CANDIDIASIS

When we think of bacteria, most of us think of something negative, such as a bacterial infection. But as I mentioned in chapter 3, bacteria are not all bad. As a matter of fact, many bacteria are very good and vitally important to the proper functioning of our bodies. On any given day, at least four hundred different varieties of bacteria—approximately a hundred trillion individual bacteria—are making residence in your GI tract. They form two different types:

- Lactobacillus acidophilus
- Bifido

These friendly bacteria live in your small and large intestines all the time, controlling mucus, debris, yeast, parasites and overgrowth of pathogenic (bad) bacteria. They also produce vitamin K and B vitamins, and they maintain the proper pH for the digestive tract.

However, if this healthy population of good bacteria is destroyed or reduced in number, your immune system and liver are forced to work much harder to deal with all the impurities and microorganisms that enter into the blood.

Friendly bacteria also neutralize toxins and cancer-causing

chemicals and prevent their absorption back into the bloodstream. Good bacteria produce lactic acid, which inhibits the growth of harmful bacteria such as salmonella, shigella, and E. coli. These good bacteria also produce fatty acids that make it difficult for candida to survive. They coat the lining of the intestines, forming a protective barrier against invasions by yeast and other microorganisms.

I start all my patients with candida on high-dose probiotics, usually 100–200 billion CFUs a day. (See Appendix B.) Listed below are medications I also recommend that will dramatically impact fatigue by eliminating candidiasis yeast.

1. *Nystatin* is a medication that has been used to treat yeast for several decades. I commonly place patients on a compounded Nystatin capsule since many of my patients have not found success trying different herbal formulas. I usually start them on two million units, three times a day.

2. *Diflucan.* If they are not improving after a month, I will usually stop the Nystatin and start them on Diflucan (100–200 mg a day) for three to six weeks. Diflucan has systemic anti-yeast properties. Before starting a systemic anti-yeast medication, I usually perform a comprehensive digestive stool analysis to determine what type of yeast a patient has and which medications or herbs the yeast responds to. I also check liver function tests before starting Diflucan and after three weeks on Diflucan.

After three to six weeks on Diflucan, I will place them back on the Nystatin or an herbal yeast formula for another two to three months or longer. (See Appendix B.) I also have them follow the candida diet and eliminate all foods they are sensitive to.

> It is useless for you to work so hard from early morning until late at night, anxiously working for food to eat; for God gives rest to his loved ones.
>
> —PSALM 127:2

A **BIBLE CURE** Prayer for You

Heavenly Father, I know that You alone can strengthen and guide me out of chronic fatigue and into Your strength and renewing power. I ask You for the wisdom to make right choices about reducing my stress, getting good nutrition, getting adequate sleep, and taking the right vitamins and supplements for my body. Thank You for the temple of my body that I can care for and use for Your glory and service. Fill me now with strength. Give me peace and rest that I may be renewed daily to live abundantly in Your good plans for my life. Amen.

A **BIBLE CURE** *Prescription*

List the vitamins you will take:

_____

_____

_____

List the supplements you need to be taking:

_____

_____

_____

List the herbs you will take:

_____

_____

_____

Complete these sentences:

The most important thing I learned about being energized with vitamins and supplements is _____

_____.

To overcome chronic fatigue, I daily need to _____

_____.

Chapter 7

REFRESH WITH THE POWER
OF SPIRITUAL JOY

H AVE YOU FELT overwhelmed by the dark weight of depression that often accompanies chronic fatigue and fibromyalgia? I have wonderful news for you. By faith you can hand that hopelessness and sadness to Jesus Christ, and in return He will refresh you with the power of spiritual joy!

If chronic fatigue or the pain of fibromyalgia overwhelms you, the cause may not be only physical. Your energy and vigor may be depleted by circumstances in your life that are taxing your energy and encumbering you. If so, turn immediately to God for strength and rest. Give your worries and cares to Him (1 Pet. 5:7).

I believe that both CFS and fibromyalgia have some underlying emotional and spiritual roots that we need to dig up and replace with the joy and gratitude that come from living a life that is fulfilling God's plan. Often, in cases of fibromyalgia, there has been a traumatic experience in a person's past, such as a physical attack or abuse, divorce, rejection, betrayal, or offense. You must identify this root and allow yourself to forgive those involved before you can "unstick" your body's stress response and begin the healing process.

Many patients have forgotten the offense and are refocused on the pain of fibromyalgia. I take these patients through forgiveness therapy, and when they cancel the debt or forgive the offense, it's like removing the thorn so the body can heal. If you have forgotten the offense, ask the Lord to search your heart according to Psalm 139:23–24 and remind you of the offense and then forgive or cancel the debt from your heart.

You might feel that you are not able to forgive those involved in hurtful situations from your past. But God's plan for you does not include living under constant stress, pain, and fatigue. God invites you to let go of the pain and bring your worries and concerns to Him in prayer. In exchange for your anxieties, He will give you peace. "Don't worry about anything; instead, pray about everything. Tell God what you need, and thank him for all he has done. Then you will experience God's peace, which exceeds anything we can understand. His peace will guard your hearts and minds as you live in Christ Jesus" (Phil. 4:6–7).

I take all of the fibromyalgia patients I treat through a process I call "forgiveness therapy." As a result, I have seen much higher success rates in treating and eliminating fibromyalgia than most other doctors or health care professionals. This is why I am so convinced that these serious emotional and spiritual issues are at the root of this painful physical condition.

Many chronic fatigue sufferers experience a great deal of sadness and even depression. The good news is that whether you are choosing to forgive some past hurts and overcome fibromyalgia or striving to conquer depression as you win the battle against chronic fatigue, a grateful heart, full of the joy of the Lord, is the biggest weapon in your arsenal. Read on for steps to help you replace the pain, sadness, and fatigue of the past with the joy of the Lord.

> The LORD is my strength and my song; he has given
> me victory. This is my God, and I will praise him—my
> father's God, and I will exalt him!
> —EXODUS 15:2

TAKE THE ONE-YEAR-TO-LIVE TEST

Suppose that you only have one year to live. What would you choose to do and not do during that time? Group these activities into three different categories:

1. The things that you enjoy doing
2. The things that you must do
3. The things that you neither enjoy nor must do

You should eliminate all of the items in category number three. For the remainder of your life, try to forget about the activities that you neither enjoy nor have to do. Do not take on any projects or commitments that may be taxing to you for the next few months until your adrenal glands become strengthened.

HIDDEN SPIRITUAL PAIN

If you're anxious, depressed, extremely angry, or grieving over a traumatic experience in your past, consider consulting professional help, such as the family doctor or a professional counselor. It is critically important to resolve these emotional conflicts in order to restore adrenal function. I recommend cognitive behavioral therapy and Thought Field Therapy to identify distortional thought processes and to resolve traumatic experiences. (See Appendix B.)

Do you have unforgiveness hidden in your heart? As I have mentioned, many chronic fatigue and fibromyalgia sufferers do. Ask the Holy Spirit to reveal to you anyone you have not forgiven, and then release them from your heart, not just from your mind.

Another thing many of the fibromyalgia patients I've treated are hiding or suppressing is rage and/or bitterness. These blocked emotions are coming out in the trigger points and muscle spasms all over their bodies, but their focus is on the pain; they are not dealing with the root of the problem, which is the rage and/or bitterness.

Do you have blocked or suppressed emotions? When you are repressing an unwanted feeling such as anger, you may not even realize it. You won't feel angry. The anger is real and explosively powerful, but it is buried deep inside the "spirit" of your mind. Your conscious mind is working hard to make you feel as if you aren't angry at all.

If you have repressed anger, you may find yourself exploding at the clerk in the grocery store because the store stopped carrying your favorite brand of bread. Or you may turn into a yelling crazy person because a little old lady cut in front of you in traffic. People with repressed anger tend to become overly agitated by seemingly insignificant things.

Rage is a powerful storm that takes few prisoners; it is a deadly force. Emotions as powerful as repressed rage (extreme, violent anger) will try to escape from the subconscious like a criminal escaping from jail. Terrible childhood traumas, including sexual, physical, verbal, and emotional abuse, can cause rage to be locked away deep inside a person's soul.

Never forget that feelings buried alive never die. Putting things out of mind doesn't eliminate them. It merely stores toxic, powerful, dangerous emotional pain—a very destructive force—deep into your subconscious. There, those feelings create great tension that eventually registers its presence in your body, especially in the trigger points of fibromyalgia.

Storing toxic emotions is like packing a closet with junk. Eventually the closet door bursts open, and everything that seemed safely hidden from view spills out on the floor.

These hidden, toxic emotions create a type of war deep within. Each time we encounter a situation that produces rage, anger, shame, or some other toxic emotion, the closet gets a little closer to bursting open. That trapped emotion actually is attempting to break into our consciousness.

The subconscious mind works harder and harder to keep it repressed, and the stress begins to produce physical symptoms in the form of muscle spasms, neck and back pain, and painful trigger points that begin to manifest in the body. Before long a vicious cycle develops. The subconscious mind continues to divert and block the conscious mind from dealing with repressed emotions, which results in tensing muscles even more, which, in turn, creates more physical pain. The fibromyalgia patient eventually becomes afraid of performing any physical activity for fear of creating more muscle tension and pain.

If you feel that what I have described as hidden spiritual pain may be expressing itself through your physical pain, be encouraged. Even if your pain has been around for many years, there's so much you can begin to do to get genuine relief from your pain. I believe that you did not pick up this Bible Cure book by accident. God sees your pain and understands it far better than you ever could. Not only does He understand you, but He is also your heavenly Father who loves you with a love that's far greater than you could ever imagine. He wants to help you uncover the roots of your pain, and He will bring lasting healing and relief.

Applying the other principles outlined in this book will doubtless provide great relief. But the most important Bible Cure step is not a physical one—it's spiritual. Why not bow your head right now and turn over your spiritual pain to Jesus? As you come to Jesus Christ, your weary soul will find rest from the raging storms of spiritual pain.

RECEIVE GOD'S WONDERFUL JOY

The wonderful joy of God's refreshing presence washes away depression, sadness, and fatigue. But the first thing you need to understand is the difference between joy and happiness.

Joy comes from within and comes from a feeling of contentment deep inside a person. It is not dependent on external circumstances but on an inner sense of purpose, fulfillment, and satisfaction.

You can choose to be joyful, or you can choose to be miserable. Joy flows from your will, and no one else can make those choices for you. Dr. Charles Swindoll once wrote, "The longer I live the more convinced I become that life is 10 percent what happens to us and 90 percent how we respond to it."[1] And we must learn to respond with joy.

The Bible gives further insight on joy:

> Always be full of joy in the Lord. I say it again—rejoice!
> —PHILIPPIANS 4:4

Rejoice is a verb that involves actions such as smiling, laughing, dancing, singing, shouting, and clapping. Rejoicing involves faith.

Happiness, on the other hand, is a feeling of pleasure that comes usually from external circumstances. It is temporary and dependent on external factors, including one's circumstances and what others say and do.

People are searching for happiness in materialism, prestige, money, careers, affairs, alcohol, gambling, drugs—but these are all happiness traps.

Sin will indeed produce happiness for a season, but it will eventually rob you of joy and peace and will lead to sorrow, insomnia, increasing stress, and eventually disease—both physical and emotional.

Joy is not going to come to you; you have to pursue and practice joy (build your joy muscles). I recommend ten belly laughs a day to all my patients. Children laugh four hundred times a day and adults only fifteen times a day,[2] but many adults get no laughter—some for years.

> A cheerful heart is good medicine.
> —PROVERBS 17:22

A **BIBLE CURE** Health Tip
Benefits of Laughter

- It relieves stress and tension, decreases stress hormones, and helps you relax.
- It improves sleep.
- It helps balance neurotransmitters, helping to relieve anxiety and depression.
- It relieves pain.
- It strengthens relationships.

- It improves the immune system.
- It's like internal jogging. One belly laugh (about twenty seconds of "guffawing") is equivalent to exercising three minutes on a rowing machine.[3]
- It may help to prevent heart attack. Research shows that people with heart disease are 40 percent less likely to laugh in various situations.[4]
- It's good for the brain and can increase problem solving and creativity.
- It increases longevity. Bob Hope and George Burns both lived to be one hundred years of age.

Most people have flabby joy muscles and bulging muscles of complaining and criticizing. To develop joy, practice what Paul tells us to do in Philippians 2:14: "Do everything without complaining and arguing." Whining, complaining people drain your energy.

Also, realize you'll never have joy if you are easily offended and bitter. That's why the apostle Paul also wrote in Ephesians 4:31–32, "Get rid of all bitterness, rage, anger, harsh words, and slander, as well as all types of evil behavior. Instead, be kind to each other, tenderhearted, forgiving one another, just as God through Christ Jesus has forgiven you."

You might be thinking, "Dr. Colbert, that's not fair!" It's not an issue of being fair but of being obedient to God's Word. Bitterness is a major cause of loss of joy and also invites mental, emotional, and physical disease, including chronic fatigue and fibromyalgia, into your body.

Forgiveness is a commandment in the Bible. It's part of the love commandment in 1 Corinthians 13: "Love keeps no record of being wronged" (v. 5). So throw away the record-keeping book.

To develop joy, change your mental software. Mark Twain said, "I've lived through some terrible things in life, some of which actually happened."[5] He was illustrating that we often perceive or remember events as being much worse than they really are. In mental health circles, this kind of thinking is called distortional thinking. You have to identify and refute distortional thought patterns if you want to develop joy in your life. Read my books *Stress Less* and *The New Bible Cure for Depression and Anxiety* for more information on distortional thinking.

The next step in developing joy is to begin to practice contentment instead of falling into the trap of materialism.

> For I have learned how to be content with whatever I have. I know how to live on almost nothing or with everything. I have learned the secret of living in every situation, whether it is with a full stomach or empty, with plenty or little.
>
> —PHILIPPIANS 4:11–12

Stop complaining about what you don't have and start being appreciative and thankful for what you have. In other words, practice gratitude. Paul writes in 1 Thessalonians 5:18, "Be thankful in all circumstances, for this is God's will for you who belong to Christ Jesus."

Practicing mindfulness increases joy and means to live in the present moment. You must slow down and do one activity at a time, bringing your full attention to the activity and your inner experience of it.

A BIBLE CURE *Health Tip*

Benefits of Gratitude

Research has found that gratitude leads to:

1. A higher income
2. Superior work outcomes—raises and promotions
3. Longer marriages
4. More friends
5. Stronger social supports and richer social interactions
6. More energy
7. Better physical health
8. A stronger immune system
9. Lower stress levels
10. A longer life (up to ten years longer in one study)[6]

God sees His character in us when we practice gratitude, and He delights in giving us the desires of our heart.

The best way to practice mindfulness is to take your child or grandchild to the park or playground and play with them. I love to take my grandson Braden to the park. He loves to play on the playground equipment, climb up the slide and slide down, swing on the swings, and play on all the equipment. But one of his favorite activities is to take tiny twigs and stick them in holes. Some of the playground equipment have a wire mesh flooring, and he will sit for an hour or more gathering twigs and sticking them through the little holes in the wire mesh flooringand watching them fall to the ground below.

In practicing mindfulness, we forget the past and future. We focus on the present moment and find something to enjoy and be grateful for in the present.

I encourage patients to make a "gratitude list." I tell them to include various parts of their body and bodily functions: eyesight; hearing; sense of smell, taste, and touch; the ability to walk. Next I ask them to list the "creature comforts" they enjoy: a hot shower, toilet, bed, refrigerator, home, car, air conditioning, food, clothing, job, and so on. Then I ask them, "How about the people in your life? List your spouse, children, family, and friends."

I'll never forget a patient I had years ago. He was dying of colon cancer and was hospitalized but so grateful. He was grateful for so many little things that you and I take for granted every day: He was thankful for someone helping him sit in a chair to look out the window. He was thankful to urinate without a catheter or bedpan. He was thankful for someone to simply turn him over in bed. He was thankful to drink cold water to soothe the sores in his mouth.

FAITH IS SO SIMPLE

Faith is not an eerie power or an extraterrestrial force. Faith is a choice. It's a choice to believe God, no matter what your circumstances and feelings may be telling you. I've traveled around the world, and I've been blessed to witness hundreds of people rising up out of wheelchairs, completely healed by God's wonderful presence (the very same presence that's with you right now). These people weren't more spiritual than you are. They weren't more religious. They didn't come from generations of preachers and saints. They were simply people who chose to believe God and believe what He said in His Book, the Bible.

Pray the following Bible Cure prayer, and then make the choice. Thank God for His wonderful promise and the incredible price

He paid to give it to you. Then thank Him continually for His incredible love for you. I join my faith with yours, and I believe together with you that the strength and comfort of the Holy Spirit are yours right now!

A **BIBLE CURE** Prayer for You

Jesus, thank You for coming in the power of God's Holy Spirit to replace my sadness with joy and my sorrow with laughter. Even if I have hidden spiritual pain, nothing is hidden from Your eyes. You see the storm in my soul. And Lord, I surrender everything that's within me right now to You. I let go of all of it and ask You to take care of it. I receive the gift of Your healing power, Your restoration, and Your salvation by faith. Thank You for Your great love for me and Your wonderful power to save me. I receive it now, in Jesus's name. Amen.

A **BIBLE CURE** *Prescription*

Do you have repressed anger, rage, or bitterness locked away in your subconscious mind? List all the people who have ever hurt or offended you, and then forgive each of them from your heart.

_____

_____

_____

Is there any hidden spiritual pain from past situations that you need to give over to God?

_____

_____

_____

If you prayed the Bible Cure prayer above, write down anything you feel God may be guiding you to do as you deal with your pain in a healthy way and break free from the grip of chronic fatigue and fibromyalgia.

_____

_____

_____

_____

FROM DON COLBERT

G OD DESIRES TO heal you of disease. His Word is full of promises that confirm His love for you and His desire to give you His abundant life. His desire includes more than physical health for you; He wants to make you whole in your mind and spirit as well through a personal relationship with His Son, Jesus Christ.

If you haven't met my best friend, Jesus, I would like to take this opportunity to introduce Him to you. It is very simple. If you are ready to let Him come into your life and become your best friend, all you need to do is sincerely pray this prayer:

> *Lord Jesus, I want to know You as my Savior and Lord. I believe You are the Son of God and that You died for my sins. I also believe You were raised from the dead and now sit at the right hand of the Father praying for me. I ask You to forgive me for my sins and change my heart so that I can be Your child and live with You eternally. Thank You for Your peace. Help me to walk with You so that I can begin to know You as my best friend and my Lord. Amen.*

If you have prayed this prayer, you have just made the most important decision of your life. I rejoice with you in your decision and your new relationship with Jesus. Please contact my publisher at pray4me@charismamedia.com so that we can send you some materials that will help you become established in your relationship with the Lord. We look forward to hearing from you.

Appendix A

CONFESSIONS FOR HEALTH AND HEALING

FIRST LET ME explain the principle of faith. Hebrews 11:6 tells us that without faith it is impossible to please God. God said, "Let the weak say, 'I am strong'" (Joel 3:10, NKJV). He didn't say let the weak talk about their weakness. We're not supposed to talk about the way we are. We are supposed to talk about the way we want to be. Get in agreement with God. I can't talk of sickness and expect health. I can't speak defeat and expect victory.

Release your faith with your words. When you speak faith, you come into agreement with God. Don't talk *about* your problems, but talk *to* your problems. When you speak about your problems, your problems *grow*; when you speak to your problems, your problems *go*.

When I say what God says about me, God has promised He will do it. Scripture says, "Let the redeemed of the LORD say so" (Ps. 107:2, NKJV). It doesn't say "think so" or "believe so." Something supernatural happens when I speak it out.

Confess the following one to two times each day.

1. I look and feel younger because God is renewing my youth. I am stronger each day and feel more energetic. Health and healing flow through me.

2. Father, I want to thank You that health and healing are flowing through my body and that sickness and disease cannot live in me.

3. I declare sickness and disease have to leave. I'm healthy and well, and God satisfies me with a long life.

4. Mountain of sickness, you must go. (It's not enough to pray or believe. You must speak to your mountain, according to Mark 11:23.)

5. Sickness, you have no right in my body. I'm a child of the most high God. I'm commanding you to leave my body.

6. God is in control. Mountain of sickness and disease, I'm saying to you, be removed. You are not in control, and you will not defeat me.

7. Sickness, you cannot stay in my life. Depression, you will not rob my joy or steal my destiny. I speak with the authority of Jesus, and all the forces of heaven come to attention. God's angels stand behind me.

8. When I face difficulties, I refuse to complain. Instead, I speak favor over my situations. When I declare favor, God will turn my mountains into molehills.

9. I have an attitude of faith, expectancy, praise, and thanksgiving.

10. I am getting healthier and healthier every day and in every way.

11. I have the mind of Christ, and the wisdom of God dwells in me. (Philippians 2:5 says, "Let this mind be in you which was also in Christ Jesus.")

12. I forgive, accept, and love myself.

13. I confess that by the stripes of Jesus I am healed (1 Pet. 2:24).

14. I boldly confess that I am healed of every disease (Ps. 103:3).

15. I am healed based on God's Word (Isa. 53:5).

16. I deny myself daily, and I give my body what it *needs* and not what it *craves*.

17. My body is not my own; it belongs to God. It is His temple, His dwelling place.

18. Whenever I feel pain and tenderness in my muscles and trigger points, the pain is simply telling my body to relax and practice belly laughter and to forgive anyone who has hurt or offended me.

19. Psalm 127:2 says that God gives His beloved sleep. I receive deep, refreshing sleep by faith, and I remain in perfect peace because my mind is stayed on the Lord (Isa. 26:3). I meditate on His Word day and night.

20. I hold fast to these confessions, and I remain in an attitude of gratitude, thanking God for restoring my health.

RESOURCES FOR CHRONIC FATIGUE AND FIBROMYALGIA

Please mention Dr. Colbert as the referring physician for the companies listed below.

Divine Health Nutritional Products
1908 Boothe Circle
Longwood, FL 32750
Phone: (407) 331-7007
Website: www.drcolbert.com
E-mail: info@drcolbert.com

Multivitamins
Divine Health Multivitamin
Divine Health Living Multivitamin

Magnesium
Divine Health Chelated Magnesium

Antioxidants
Divine Health Living CoQ10
Divine Health PQQ Plus

Glutathione-Boosting Supplements
Max One (Best for Chronic Fatigue and Fibromyalgia)
Max ATP (Best for Chronic Fatigue and Fibromyalgia)
Max GXL

D-Ribose
Divine Health Enhanced D-Ribose

Hormone Support
Divine Health Natural Progesterone Cream

Sleep
Divine Health Melatonin
Divine Health Serotonin Max (for sleep or depression)
Divine Health L-Theanine

Candida Support
Divine Health Yeast Formula
Divine Health Probiotic

Adaptogens
Divine Health Stress Manager

Muscle Spasms With Fibromyalgia
Divine Health FM Formula (Fibromyalgia Formula) (Malic acid and magnesium)

Supplements From Don Colbert, MD
1908 Boothe Circle
Longwood, FL 32750
Phone: (407) 331-7007

Mitochondrial Basics With PQQ (acetyl L-carnitine, alpha lipoic acid, and PQQ)
GABA
Tryptopure (L-trypotphan)
Stress Relief Drops
Theralac (Probiotic with 30 billion colony forming units)

Probiomax (Probiotic with 50 billion colony forming units)

Saccharomycin DF (Probiotic with 5 billion colony forming units)

Adrenal Support (Adrenal rebuilder and adrenal glandular)

Pregnenolone PleoLyposome Cream

DHEA PleoLyposome Cream

Corticare B (High dose vitamin B_5)

B Complex Plus

Fulvic Minerals

Food Sensitivities

Sage Medical Laboratory

Phone: (877) SAGE LAB

Website: www.sagemedlab.com

Thought Field Therapy

Callahan Techniques

Website: www.rogercallahan.com

Cognitive-Behavioral Therapy

Website: www.nacbt.org

From the health food store

Sleepy Time Tea, Sleepy Time Tea Extra, Bedtime Tea, Chamomile Tea, NADH, Natrol Melatonin sublingual (Wal-Mart)

To find a doctor to prescribe bioidentical hormones, Myer's IV and medications for candida, including Nystatin and Diflucan:

Web site: www.worldhealth.com

Mercury and Heavy Metal Detox

Refer to www.autismpedia.org, ALA/DMSA Mercury Detoxification Protocol by Andrew Hall Cutler, PhD, PE

Igenex Lyme Disease Test

Website: www.igenex.com

NOTES

INTRODUCTION
A BRAND-NEW BIBLE CURE FOR A BRAND-NEW YOU!

1. K. Kimberly McCleary and Suzanne D. Vernon, "Chronic Fatigue Syndrome," *The Pain Practitioner* 20, no. 1 (Spring 2010): 14–19, http://www.cfids.org/about-cfids/pain-practitioner-spring2010.pdf (accessed March 23, 2011).

2. DePaul University, "The CFIDS Association of America Applauds Research Presenting Clearer Picture of Chronic Fatigue Syndrome," press release, October 7, 1999, http://condor.depaul.edu/ljason/cfs/press.html (accessed March 23, 2011), referencing upcoming publication of Leonard A. Jason et al., "A Community-Based Study of Chronic Fatigue Syndrome," *Archives of Internal Medicine* 159, no. 18 (October 11, 1999): 2129–2137, http://archinte.ama-assn.org/cgi/content/full/159/18/2129 (accessed March 23, 2011).

CHAPTER 1
UNDERSTANDING CHRONIC FATIGUE AND FIBROMYALGIA

1. Jason et al., "A Community-Based Study of Chronic Fatigue Syndrome."

2. McCleary and Vernon, "Chronic Fatigue Syndrome."

CHAPTER 2
UNCOVERING THE CAUSES OF AND CONTRIBUTING FACTORS TO CHRONIC FATIGUE AND FIBROMYALGIA

1. Kirk Stokel, "Rejuvenate Your Cells by Growing Mitochondria," *Life Extension* 2010/2011, http://www.lef.org/magazine/mag2010/ss2010_Rejuvenate-Your-Cells-Growing-New-Mitochondria_01.htm (accessed March 21, 2011).

2. American Psychological Association, "Why Sleep Is Important and What Happens When You Don't Get Enough," http://www.apa.org/topics/sleep/why.aspx (accessed March 23, 2011).

3. ScienceDaily.com, "New Study Shows Sinus Surgery Can Improve Chronic Fatigue," November 2, 2004, http://www.sciencedaily.com/releases/2004/10/041030212628.htm (accessed December 13, 2010).

4. Deirder Imus, "The Danger Lurking in Compact Fluorescent Light Bulbs," FoxNews.com, March 7, 2011, http://www.foxnews.com/health/2011/03/07/danger-lurking-compact-fluorescent-light-bulbs/ (accessed March 17, 2011).

5. Leigh Erin Connealy, "The Mad Hatter Syndrome: Mercury and Biological Toxicity," NaturalNews.com, January 6, 2006, http://www.naturalnews.com/016544.html (accessed March 24, 2011).

6. Gina Shaw, "Mercury Fillings the Hidden Cause of Chronic Fatigue and Other Illnesses?", Wisconsin ME/CFS Association, Inc., http://www.wicfs-me.org/mercury_cause_cfs.htm (accessed December 15, 2010).

7. FDA.gov, "Mercury Levels in Commercial Fish and Shellfish," November 19, 2009, http://www.fda.gov/food/foodsafety/product-specificinformation/seafood/foodbornepathogenscontaminants/methylmercury/ucm115644.htm (accessed March 24, 2011).

CHAPTER 3
REFUEL WITH NUTRITION

1. George M. Wolverton, "Xanthines (the Evils of)," 21st Century Medicine newsletter, http://www.21stcenturymed.net/newsletters/xanthines.htm (accessed February 1, 2011).

2. National Academy of Sciences, "Antibiotic Use in Food Animals Contributes to Microbe Resistance," news release, July 9, 1998, http://www8.nationalacademies.org/onpinews/newsitem.aspx?RecordID=5137 (accessed March 24, 2011).

CHAPTER 4
RECHARGE WITH EXERCISE

1. Albert E. Carter, *Rebound Exercise: The Ultimate Exercise for the New Millennium* (Bloomington, IN: AuthorHouse, 2006), 15–16.

CHAPTER 5
RENEW WITH REST

1. Center for Science in the Public Interest, "Caffeine Content of Food and Drugs," September 2007, http://www.cspinet.org/new/cafchart.htm (accessed March 24, 2011).

2. SleepMed.com, "Sleep Statistics," http://sleepmed.me/page/1896 (accessed May 5, 2011).

CHAPTER 6
RESTORE WITH VITAMINS AND SUPPLEMENTS

1. ChronicFatigueTreatments.com, "Glutathione and Chronic Fatigue Syndrome," *Chronic Fatigue* (blog), February 10, 2007, http://www.chronicfatiguetreatments.com/wordpress/treatments/glutathione-and-chronic-fatigue-syndrome/ (accessed January 26, 2011).

2. P. C. Tullson and R. L. Terjung, "Adenine Nucleotide Synthesis in Exercising and Endurance-Trained Skeletal Muscle," *American Journal of Physiology* 261, no. 2 (C342–C347), referenced in Julius G. Goepp, "Rejuvenate Cardiac Cellular Energy Production," LifeExtensionVitamins.com, May 2008, http://www.lifeextensionvitamins.com/may08denyohe.html (accessed March 24, 2011).

CHAPTER 7
REFRESH WITH THE POWER OF SPIRITUAL JOY

1. Charles R. Swindoll, *Strengthening Your Grip* (Nashville: Thomas Nelson, 1990), 206.

2. Doug Dvorak, "A Laugh a Day Keeps the Doctor Away—Laugh Your Way Back to Health," eZineArticles.com, http://ezinearticles.com/?A-Laugh-A-Day-Keeps-The-Doctor-Away---Laugh-Your-Way-Back-To-Health&id=323872 (accessed March 25, 2011).

3. Janice Norris, "Laughter Is Good Medicine," *Health Is Wealth* (blog), *The Sun Times*, March 23, 2011, http://www.thesuntimes.com/newsnow/x13293848/Laughter-is-good-medicine (accessed March 25, 2011).

4. University of Maryland Medical Center, "Laughter Is Good for Your Heart, According to a New University of Maryland Medical Center Study," news release, November 15, 2000, http://www.umm.edu/news/releases/laughter.htm (accessed March 28, 2011).

5. GoodReads.com, "Mark Twain Quotes," http://www.goodreads.com/author/quotes/1655.Mark_Twain (accessed March 25, 2011).

6. D. D. Danner, D. Snowden, and W. V. Friesen, "Positive Emotions in Early Life and Longevity: Findings From the Nun Study," *Journal of Personality and Social Psychology* 80 (2001): 804–813, referenced in Charles D. Kerns, "Gratitude at Work," *Graziadio Business Review* 9, no. 4 (2006), http://gbr.pepperdine.edu/064/quote/17764/ (accessed March 25, 2011).

Don Colbert, MD, was born in Tupelo, Mississippi. He attended Oral Roberts School of Medicine in Tulsa, Oklahoma, where he received a bachelor of science degree in biology in addition to his degree in medicine. Dr. Colbert completed his internship and residency with Florida Hospital in Orlando, Florida. He is board certified in family practice and anti-aging medicine and has received extensive training in nutritional medicine.

If you would like more information about natural and divine healing, or information about ***Divine Health nutritional products,*** you may contact Dr. Colbert at:

DON COLBERT, MD
1908 Boothe Circle
Longwood, FL 32750
Telephone: 407-331-7007 (for ordering products only)
Website: www.drcolbert.com.

Disclaimer: Dr. Colbert and the staff of Divine Health Wellness Center are prohibited from addressing a patient's medical condition by phone, facsimile, or e-mail. Please refer questions related to your medical condition to your own primary care physician.

Pick up these great Bible Cure books by Don Colbert, MD:

The Bible Cure for ADD and Hyperactivity
The Bible Cure for Allergies
The Bible Cure for Arthritis
The Bible Cure for Asthma
The Bible Cure for Autoimmune Diseases
The Bible Cure for Back Pain
The Bible Cure for Candida and Yeast Infections
The Bible Cure for Colds, Flu and Sinus Infections
The Bible Cure for Headaches
The Bible Cure for Heartburn and Indigestion
The Bible Cure for Hepatitis and Hepatitis C
The Bible Cure for High Blood Pressure
The Bible Cure for High Cholesterol
The Bible Cure for Irritable Bowel Syndrome
The Bible Cure for Memory Loss
The Bible Cure for Menopause
The Bible Cure for PMS and Mood Swings
The Bible Cure for Prostate Disorders
The Bible Cure for Skin Disorders
The Bible Cure for Thyroid Disorders
The Bible Cure for Weight Loss and Muscle Gain
The Bible Cure Recipes for Overcoming Candida
The New Bible Cure for Chronic Fatigue and Fibromyalgia
The New Bible Cure for Depression and Anxiety
The New Bible Cure for Diabetes
The New Bible Cure for Cancer
The New Bible Cure for Heart Disease
The New Bible Cure for Osteoporosis
The New Bible Cure for Sleep Disorders
The New Bible Cure for Stress

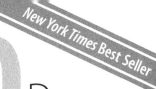
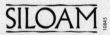